Physical Examination of the Spine

Second Edition

Todd J. Albert, MD
Surgeon-in-Chief
Medical Director
Korein-Wilson Professor of Orthopaedic Surgery
Hospital for Special Surgery
Chairman
Department of Orthopaedic Surgery
Weill Cornell Medical College
New York, New York

Alexander R. Vaccaro, MD, PhD, MBA
Richard H. Rothman Professor and Chairman
Department of Orthopaedic Surgery
Professor of Neurosurgery
Thomas Jefferson University and Hospitals
President
The Rothman Institute
Philadelphia, Pennsylvania

213 illustrations

Thieme
New York • Stuttgart • Delhi • Rio de Janeiro

Executive Editor: William Lamsback
Managing Editor: Sarah Landis
Director, Editorial Services: Mary Jo Casey
Editorial Assistant: Nikole Connors
Production Editor: Naamah Schwartz
International Production Director:
    Andreas Schabert
Vice President, Editorial and E-Product
    Development: Vera Spillner
International Marketing Director: Fiona Henderson
International Sales Director: Louisa Turrell
Director of Sales, North America: Mike Roseman
Senior Vice President and Chief Operating Officer:
    Sarah Vanderbilt
President: Brian D. Scanlan

Library of Congress Cataloging-in-Publication Data

Names: Albert, Todd J., author. | Vaccaro, Alexander R., author.
Title: Physical examination of the spine / Todd J. Albert, Alexander R. Vaccaro.
Description: Second edition. | New York : Thieme, [2017] | Includes bibliographical references and index.
Identifiers: LCCN 2016036778| ISBN 9781626233201 (hardcover) | ISBN 9781626233218 (eISBN)
Subjects: | MESH: Spine | Physical Examination--methods | Spinal
    Diseases—diagnosis
Classification: LCC RD768 | NLM WE 725 | DDC 616.7/3075—dc23
LC record available at https://lccn.loc.gov/2016036778

Important note: Medicine is an ever-changing science undergoing continual development. Research and clinical experience are continually expanding our knowledge, in particular our knowledge of proper treatment and drug therapy. Insofar as this book mentions any dosage or application, readers may rest assured that the authors, editors, and publishers have made every effort to ensure that such references are in accordance with **the state of knowledge at the time of production of the book.**

Nevertheless, this does not involve, imply, or express any guarantee or responsibility on the part of the publishers in respect to any dosage instructions and forms of applications stated in the book. **Every user is requested to examine carefully** the manufacturers' leaflets accompanying each drug and to check, if necessary in consultation with a physician or specialist, whether the dosage schedules mentioned therein or the contraindications stated by the manufacturers differ from the statements made in the present book. Such examination is particularly important with drugs that are either rarely used or have been newly released on the market. Every dosage schedule or every form of application used is entirely at the user's own risk and responsibility. The authors and publishers request every user to report to the publishers any discrepancies or inaccuracies noticed. If errors in this work are found after publication, errata will be posted at www.thieme.com on the product description page.

Some of the product names, patents, and registered designs referred to in this book are in fact registered trademarks or proprietary names even though specific reference to this fact is not always made in the text. Therefore, the appearance of a name without designation as proprietary is not to be construed as a representation by the publisher that it is in the public domain.

© 2017 Thieme Medical Publishers, Inc.

Thieme Publishers New York
333 Seventh Avenue, New York, NY 10001 USA
+1 800 782 3488, customerservice@thieme.com

Thieme Publishers Stuttgart
Rüdigerstrasse 14, 70469 Stuttgart, Germany
+49 [0]711 8931 421, customerservice@thieme.de

Thieme Publishers Delhi
A-12, Second Floor, Sector-2, Noida-201301
Uttar Pradesh, India
+91 120 45 566 00, customerservice@thieme.in

Thieme Publishers Rio de Janeiro, Thieme Publicações Ltda.
Edifício Rodolpho de Paoli, 25º andar
Av. Nilo Peçanha, 50 – Sala 2508
Rio de Janeiro 20020-906 Brasil
+55 21 3172-2297 / +55 21 3172-1896

Cover design: Thieme Publishing Group
Typesetting by DiTech Process Solutions

Printed in China by Everbest Printing Co.   5 4 3 2 1

ISBN 978-1-62623-320-1

Also available as an e-book:
eISBN 978-1-62623-321-8

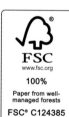

FSC
www.fsc.org
100%
Paper from well-managed forests
FSC® C124385

Contents

Preface

Since the publication of the first edition of *Physical Examination of the Spine*, spinal diagnostics and evaluations and technology have continued to progress at a rapid rate. Multiple scanning techniques, diagnostic modalities, and technologies to aid in diagnosis have continued to improve and become ever more sophisticated. Even with the fast pace of technological advancement, nothing can replace a good history and physical examination to help with diagnosis and ultimately creation of a treatment plan to help our patients. This is important not only for students and residents in all medical specialties, but also for physical therapists, physician assistants, and nurses in order to understand that which is ailing our patients. It continues to be our hope that this book will help all of these providers to understand and improve their spinal diagnostic capabilities through well-executed and comprehensive physical examination.

The history continues to be the first opportunity the healthcare provider has to understand the patient's problem in that it helps direct a more systems-focused physical examination. This is especially important in patients with spinal disorders where history can help exclude causes of disability that may not be spine-related but also alert us to red flags that may indicate more immediate advanced spinal imaging. Spinal stenosis is an excellent example. If the patient presents with a complaint of difficulty and leg pain that occurred when walking and difficulty ambulating when erect which is relieved with sitting, it can either be neurogenic claudication caused by nerve compression or vascular claudication. If the patient is able to sit and ride a bike endlessly without causing the pain, it is more likely spinal stenosis as opposed to vascular claudication. Additionally, if the patient presents with significant back pain but on history is found to have pain that wakes them at night and/or a history of fever, chills, or weight loss, this may imply either an infection or malignant condition that requires workup with laboratory studies and advanced imaging.

The book is again divided into anatomic regions of the spine—cervical, thoracic and lumbosacral—and has anatomical structures identified for ease of understanding. New to this edition are color illustrations that will make the examples more clear and precise. We have continued to include a special section on spinal deformity as this has been lacking in other books; this was included in our first edition and enhanced in this edition. We hope that this book will continue to be helpful as a reference for the practicing physician as well as the first-time student trying to understand and learn physical diagnosis.

In a world of increasing complexity in healthcare, delivery of healthcare and in diagnostics, we hope that this book continues to serve as a basis for the most important diagnostic testing we do for our patients—the history and physical examination. We also hope that it will continue to improve the quality of care you are able to offer your patients.

Todd J. Albert, MD

Alexander R. Vaccaro, MD, PhD, MBA

Acknowledgments and Dedication

We want to acknowledge and thank Daniel Stein, who has helped tremendously in the editing and creation of this second edition of *Physical Examination of the Spine*. He worked tirelessly to enhance this new edition from the first, identifying important components of the text that were worthy of further refinement.

Our deepest appreciation for his efforts.

Todd J. Albert, MD
Alexander R. Vaccaro, MD, PhD, MBA

Chapter 1

The Fundamentals

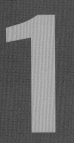

1 The Fundamentals

Accurate diagnosis of spinal disease requires a thorough history, physical examination, and analysis of appropriate imaging studies, when necessary. Often, the most important priority is to rule out alternative disease processes that can mimic spinal disorders. To accomplish these goals, a comprehensive understanding of basic spinal/neural anatomy is necessary as a first step.

■ Basic Anatomy of the Spine

The vertebral column consists of 33 vertebrae, divided into 5 segments: cervical, thoracic, lumbar, sacral, and coccygeal (**Fig. 1.1**). There are 7 cervical, 12 thoracic, 5 lumbar, 5 sacral, and 4 coccygeal vertebrae. The sacral and coccygeal vertebrae are usually fused to form the sacrum and the coccyx, respectively. The vertebrae of each segment are similar with several variations. The typical vertebra consists of a body, spinous process, two transverse processes, two pedicles, two arches, and two laminae (**Fig. 1.2**).

The two major exceptions are C1 and C2 (**Fig. 1.3a, b**). The first cervical vertebra, C1, is called the atlas and lacks the vertebral body. The atlas forms the atlanto-occipital joint with the occiput of the skull and contributes to flexion and extension of the neck (**Fig. 1.3c**). The second cervical vertebra is called the axis. Located on the superior side of the body of C2 is a bony protrusion called the dens or odontoid process. The dens fits into the ring of the atlas. Together, the atlas and axis make up the atlantoaxial joint, the major contributor to cervical rotation. The vertebral bodies between C2 and S1 are separated from each other by fibrocartilaginous intervertebral disks that act as buffers to mechanical shocks.

The spinal cord resides within the vertebral foramen and extends from C1 to its ending, the conus medullaris, between L1 and L2 (**Fig. 1.4**). The filum terminale extends from the conus medullaris and attaches to the coccyx. The spinal cord is segmented, and 1 of the 31 pairs of spinal nerves exits from each segment of the spinal cord. There are 8 cervical, 12 thoracic, 5 lumbar, and 5 sacral pairs, and 1 coccygeal pair of spinal nerves. The spinal nerves of the cervical, thoracic, and lumbar cord exit through the intervertebral foramina; the sacral spinal nerves make up the cauda equina and exit through the sacral foramina.

■ Basic Neurology of the Spine

The spinal cord consists of a cellular core called gray matter surrounded by a fibrous layer called white matter. Spinal neurons, known as lower motor neurons, and interneurons reside in the gray matter. The axons of lower motor neurons together with afferent sensory neuron axons make up the white matter. The white matter is divided into four funiculi: right lateral, left lateral, ventral, and dorsal. Within the white matter are tracts of ascending and descending axons segregated into pathways of function (**Fig. 1.5**). Some of the most useful diagnostic pathways are the lateral spinothalamic tract, the dorsal columns, and the lateral corticospinal tracts.

The lateral spinothalamic tract mediates pain and temperature sensation. The tract crosses the cord at the level of entry and ascends to the brain in the lateral funiculus. A unilateral injury to the lateral spinothalamic tract will therefore result in a loss of pain and temperature on the contralateral side (**Fig. 1.6a**).

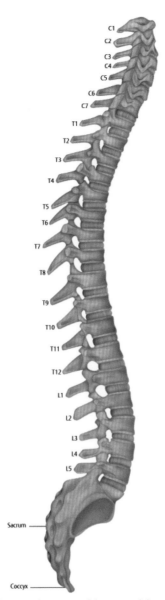

C1
C2
C3
C4
C5
C6
C7
T1
T2
T3
T4
T5
T6
T7
T8
T9
T10
T11
T12
L1
L2
L3
L4
L5
Sacrum
Coccyx

Fig. 1.1 Normal sagittal alignment and bony architecture of the cervical thoracic, lumbar, and sacrococcygeal spine.

The dorsal column pathway mediates vibration sensation, two-point touch, and conscious proprioception. The dorsal column pathway ascends in the ipsilateral dorsal funiculus until decussation in the brainstem. A unilateral injury to the dorsal funiculus (**Fig. 1.6b**) will therefore result in a loss of vibration sensation, two-point touch, and conscious proprioception on the same side.

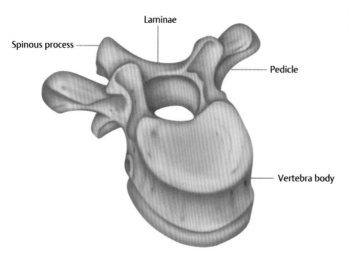

Fig. 1.2 Normal vertebra with body, processes, pedicles, and laminae.

Laminae

Spinous process

Pedicle

Vertebra body

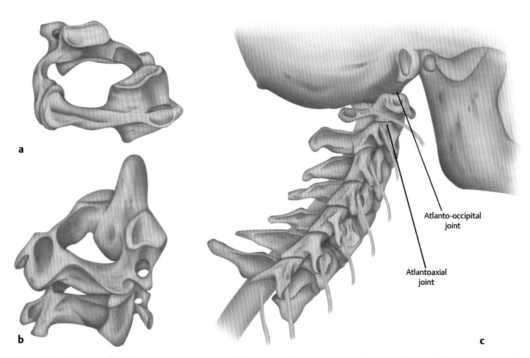

a

b

c

Atlanto-occipital joint

Atlantoaxial joint

Fig. 1.3 (**a**) C1 and (**b**) C2 vertebrae. Note the difference in these two vertebrae, with the C1 being a ring and the C2 forming a bony peg that articulates with the ring of C1. (**c**) The atlantoaxial and atlanto-occipital joints contribute significantly to rotation and flexion/extension of the skull on the neck.

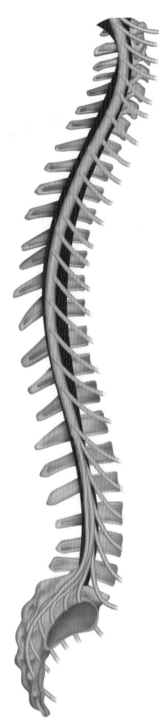

Fig. 1.4 The neural anatomy is such that the spinal cord resides within the bony canal between C1 and L1 and/or L2. The filum terminale extends from the conus and attaches to the coccyx.

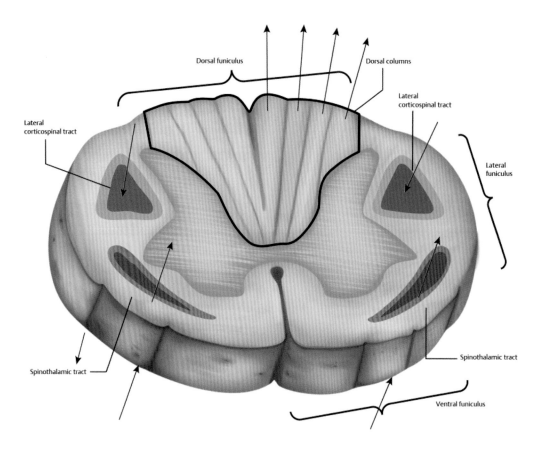

Fig. 1.5 Cross section of the spinal cord delineating white and gray matter and four funiculi.

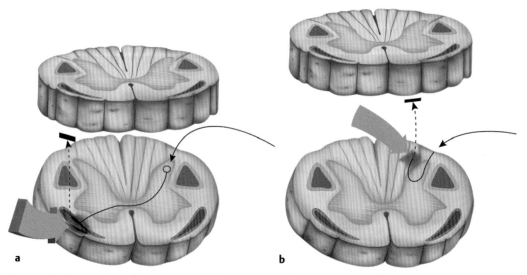

Fig. 1.6 (a) Cross section of the spinal cord delineating the spinothalamic tract. (b) Cross section of the spinal cord delineating the dorsal column.

The lateral corticospinal tract mediates voluntary motor function. The tract descends in the lateral funiculus to interneurons and lower motor neurons residing in the gray matter. The lateral corticospinal tract initially crosses in the brainstem and descends the spinal cord on the contralateral side to its origin in the brain. The descending tract in the cord is ipsilateral to the muscle it mediates. A unilateral lesion to the lateral funiculus will therefore result in a loss of function on the ipsilateral side.

A lesion to the lateral corticospinal tract is called an upper motor neuron lesion and results in spastic paralysis. Upper motor neurons synapse on lower motor neurons and interneurons to modulate their activity. The majority of the signals sent by upper motor neurons are inhibitory. When the axons of the upper motor neurons are lesioned, the modulation on the lower motor neurons is released, and they fire at will. This results in spastic paralysis. In contrast, a lesion to a peripheral nerve or damage to lower motor neuron cell bodies results in flaccid paralysis.

■ Sensation Testing

Sensory testing is broken down into several different modalities. These include temperature (**Fig. 1.7**), two-point discrimination, sharp versus dull pain, vibration (**Fig. 1.8**), and the ability to distinguish between light and deep pressure. When grading the sensory examination, each test should be performed consecutively on alternating sides of the body to allow direct comparison between sensations on each side. Patients should be instructed to close their eyes or look away when testing.

Sharp Sensation

The sharp sensation (pain) is tested with a pin. To perform the exam properly, the examiner must elicit pain and not pressure. To do this, the pin must be pushed firmly onto the skin (taking care not to perforate the surface). The patient should compare the intensity of the sensation on both sides.

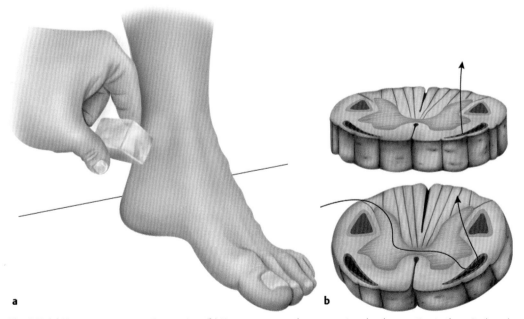

a   b

Fig. 1.7 (**a**) Temperature sensation testing. (**b**) Temperature pathway crossing the decussation in the spinal cord.

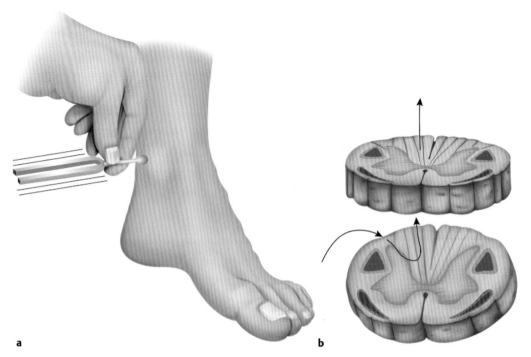

Fig. 1.8 (**a**) Testing vibration sensation, a dorsal column function. (**b**) Pathway of vibration sensation.

Temperature

Temperature sensation is most commonly tested using a cold object (**Fig. 1.7a**). An ice cube or alcohol pad may be used, but more often the handle of a reflex hammer is sufficient. The test is performed by pressing the cold object onto various locations on the patient's skin. The patient's ability to detect cold is noted, as well as any changes in the degree of perception.

Two-Point Discrimination

Two-point discrimination is tested with two sharp, fine objects. Pins are commonly used. The pins are lightly pushed against the skin and brought repeatedly closer together until the patient can no longer feel two separate points of contact. Different areas of the body will yield different results; the test should therefore be compared with the test at the same location on the opposite side.

Sharp versus Dull Sensation

Strict attention must be paid to the patient's discrimination between sharp and dull sensation. The tip and head of the pin can be used. Each one is pushed against the skin, and the patient is asked to determine if the object is sharp or dull. The patient should be instructed to look away or close the eyes.

Vibration

Vibration testing is best performed by placing the end of a tuning fork on bony structures (**Fig. 1.8a**). The medial and lateral malleoli, as well as the styloid processes of the radius and ulna, are common locations for testing vibratory sensation.

Light versus Deep Pressure

Pressure testing is best performed by pressing a fine, dull object onto the skin (the head of a pin may be used). With the patient's eyes closed, the object is pressed lightly onto the skin, first with light and then with deep pressure. The patient is asked to describe any difference in sensation.

■ Muscle Testing

The techniques of muscle testing are specific to each exam and are discussed in Chapters 2 to 4. Consistency in testing is extremely important, and the same examiner should test the patient over time for the best evaluation. It is extremely important that maximum effort be exerted during testing to elucidate subtle muscle weakness, which can be clinically important.

■ Muscle Grading

The grading system most commonly used to communicate muscle strength is as follows:

- Grade 0 (no function): Total paralysis.
- Grade 1 (trace): Palpable or visual contraction without joint motion.
- Grade 2 (poor): Complete range of motion of joint with gravity eliminated.
- Grade 3 (fair): Complete range of motion of joint against gravity.
- Grade 4 (good): Complete range of motion of joint against gravity with some resistance.
- Grade 5 (normal): Complete range of motion of joint against gravity and resistance (unbreakable).
- Half grades (i.e., --, -, +, ++) are occasionally used in clinical conversation.

■ Classifications of Muscle Grading

Other classifications of grading are sometimes used, such as the Frankel classification,[1] the Bradford and McBride division of the Frankel classification,[2] the American Spinal Injury Association (ASIA) Impairment Scale, or one of the many other classification systems that are not discussed in this book.

Frankel Classification System (for Spinal Cord Injury)

- Frankel A: No motor or sensory function
- Frankel B: No motor function, sensory incomplete
- Frankel C: Motor function useless, sensory incomplete
- Frankel D: Motor function useful, sensory incomplete
- Frankel E: Motor function normal, sensory normal

Bradford and McBride Divisions of Frankel D

- Frankel D1: Preserved motor function at lowest functional grade with or without bowel and bladder paralysis with normal or reduced voluntary motor function
- Frankel D2: Preserved motor function at midfunctional grade and normal voluntary bowel or bladder function.
- Frankel D3: Preserved motor function at high functional grade and normal voluntary bowel and bladder function.

American Spinal Injury Association Impairment Scale

- A (complete): No motor or sensory function is preserved in the sacral segments S4–S5.
- B (incomplete): Sensory but not motor function is preserved below the neurologic level of injury and extends through the sacral segments S4–S5.
- C (incomplete): Motor function is preserved below the neurologic level of injury, and the majority of key muscles below that level have a muscle grade less than 3 (nonuseful function).
- D (incomplete): Motor function is preserved below the neurologic level of injury, and a majority of key muscles below the neurologic level have a muscle grade greater than or equal to 3.
- E (normal): Motor and sensory function is normal.

■ Reflex Testing

Reflex testing, like muscle testing, relies on consistency in grading. The same examiner should therefore conduct all of the testing when applicable. If the patient is concentrating on the reflex response and interfering with the results, the examiner may wish to create a distraction by asking the patient to lock the hands and pull them apart. The specific testing will be delineated in the following chapters.

■ Reflex Grading Classification System

The reflex classification system is as follows:

- Grade 0: No reflex
- Grade 1: Slight response
- Grade 2: Normal reflex
- Grade 3: Hyperactive
- Grade 4: Hyperactive with clonus
- Half grades (i.e., --, -, +, ++) can be used occasionally in clinical conversation

The reflex response may differ with age. A normal child may classify as a 4 on this scale when compared with an average adult. A normal elderly man may have a response of 1.

References

1. Frankel HL, Hancock GH, Melzak J, et al. The value of postural reduction in the initial management of closed injuries of the spine with paraplegia and tetraplegia. I. Paraplegia 1969;73:179–192
2. Bradford DS, McBride GG. Surgical management of thoracolumbar spine fractures with incomplete neurologic deficits. Clin Orthop Relat Res 1987;(218):201–216

Chapter 2

Physical Examination of the Cervical Spine

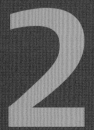

2 Physical Examination of the Cervical Spine

The cervical spine exam is particularly important in patients with axial neck pain, arm pain, neurologic dysfunction of the upper or lower extremities, or bowel and/or bladder dysfunction. Because all of these symptoms can emanate from pathologies related to the cervical spine, spinal cord, or nerve roots, questions related to these types of symptoms should be posed while taking a history. Care should be taken to rule out myelopathy (signs/symptoms of spinal cord compression) to allow the patient an understanding of the risks associated with cervical spinal cord compression. If the patient has radicular complaints (pain, sensory changes, or weakness in a nerve root distribution), it behooves the examiner to try to delineate which nerve root is affected during the history and physical examination. Finally, always ask pertinent questions to help rule out a tumor or infection (night pain, fevers, chills, sweats, or unexplained weight loss).

■ Inspection

Visual Inspection

Patient inspection starts when the patient enters the room. Observe the patient's attitude. Note if the patient is in pain, irritated, angry, or frustrated, and if the complaint is a possible cause. Pay particular attention to see if the patient is protecting (splinting) any part of the body. Observe how the patient carries the head. Watch the patient, and note any kyphosis (hunchback), scoliosis (S-shaped curve), torticollis (twisted neck), difference in shoulder height, or other abnormalities. If the patient presents with an abnormality in posture, determine whether the patient can correct it without assistance. Be sure to note any pain. Try to deduce if the patient's positioning could be causing the problem, and attempt to determine its relation to the patient's complaint.

Much can be learned from observing the patient undress. Motion of the head and neck normally should be smooth and fluid. Notice if the patient is limited in any motions or has trouble pulling the shirt over the head, unbuttoning buttons, or bending to take off shoes and socks. Note the patient's range of motion and amount of pain. Once the patient is undressed, look for any signs of trauma, blisters, scars, discoloration, contusions, limb asymmetry, and atrophy.

Palpation

Before palpating, you may wish first to check for variation in skin temperature and for diaphoresis by comparing symptomatic with asymptomatic areas using the back of the hand. Marked changes in temperature may indicate to the examiner areas where care should be taken not to cause unnecessary pain during palpation. Perform palpation systematically, using first bony and then soft tissue. When palpating the bony structures, note any asymmetries, misalignments, lumps, abnormalities, and areas of tenderness. In soft tissue palpation, take note of tension and tenderness of the skin; the size, shape, and firmness of the muscles and any masses; and any other asymmetric differences found during the exam. Try to differentiate recent soft tissue changes that feel softer and more tender from older changes that will feel harder and more stringy. In addition, pay particular attention to the peripheral pulse; low pulse rate with low blood pressure could be the result of a sympathectomy from a spinal cord injury.

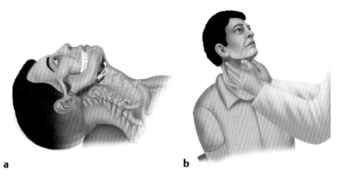

Fig. 2.1 (**a**) Position of the patient in extension for palpation of the anterior cervical spine. (**b**) Position of the patient in the seated position for palpation of the anterior cervical spine.

a
b

Palpation of the Anterior Cervical Spine

The anterior cervical spine can be palpated while the patient is sitting or in the supine position (**Fig. 2.1a, b**). Positioning of the patient should be determined by patient comfort, rather than the preference of the medical professional. If the patient is more comfortable in the sitting position, the examiner should stand in front of the patient. If the patient wishes to be examined while lying down, the examiner should stand near/towards the head of the patient. For palpation in either of these positions, the examiner should stand at the patient's side, place one hand under the patient's neck for support, and use the other for palpation. The examination of the anterior cervical spine should begin with bony structure and cartilaginous tissue palpation. Important structures to assess include the hyoid bone, the thyroid cartilage, the first cricoid ring, the trachea, and the carotid tubercle. Follow this with soft tissue palpation, which consists of the sternocleidomastoid muscle and associated lymph nodes (looking for adenopathy), the carotid pulse, the parotid gland, and the supraclavicular fossa (**Fig. 2.2**).

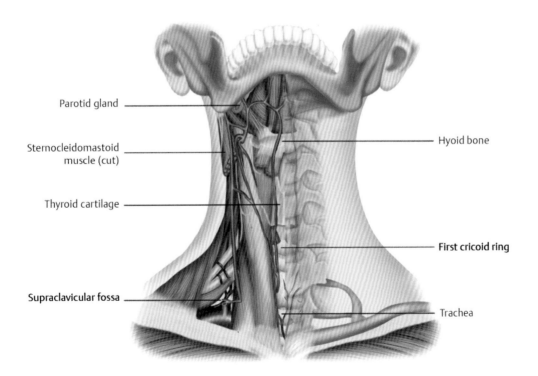

Parotid gland

Sternocleidomastoid muscle (cut)

Thyroid cartilage

Supraclavicular fossa

Hyoid bone

First cricoid ring

Trachea

Fig. 2.2 Anterior view of the cervical spine, with muscular anatomy on the left and bony anatomy on the right.

Bony and Cartilaginous Structure Palpation of the Anterior Cervical Spine

Hyoid Bone

Palpation: The hyoid bone is a horseshoe-shaped structure opening toward the spine. It is palpable by placing the thumb and index finger on each side of the neck, above the thyroid cartilage and below the mandible (**Fig. 2.3**). Ask the patient to swallow, and feel for the hyoid bone as it elevates. Take care when palpating the hyoid bone because moderate pressure may cause it to break. The hyoid bone lies in a horizontal plane at the level of the C3 vertebral body.

Thyroid Cartilage and Thyroid Gland

Palpation: Begin by locating the thyroid cartilage. Start high in the midline of the anterior neck, and palpate inferiorly until you feel its superior notch (**Fig. 2.4**). The prominent, superior portion of the thyroid cartilage, commonly known as the Adam's apple (**Fig. 2.5**), lies in a horizontal plane with the C4 vertebral body. The inferior portion of the thyroid cartilage lies in a plane horizontal with the C5 vertebral body. Lateral and posterior to the thyroid cartilage is the thyroid gland (**Fig. 2.6**). Palpate the thyroid gland on both sides.
  Findings: A normal thyroid gland should be symmetric and smooth. If the gland feels cystic or lumpy, further work-up may be necessary to rule out disease of the thyroid.

First Cricoid Ring

Palpation: The first cricoid ring is located just below the thyroid cartilage (**Fig. 2.7**). Ask the patient to swallow; this will cause the first cricoid ring to elevate and will make palpation easier. The first cricoid ring lies in a horizontal plane with the C6 vertebral body. Take care when palpating the cricoid cartilage; too much pressure may cause the patient to gag.

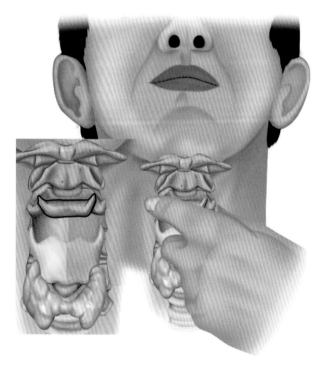

Fig. 2.3 Palpation of the hyoid bone in the anterior neck.

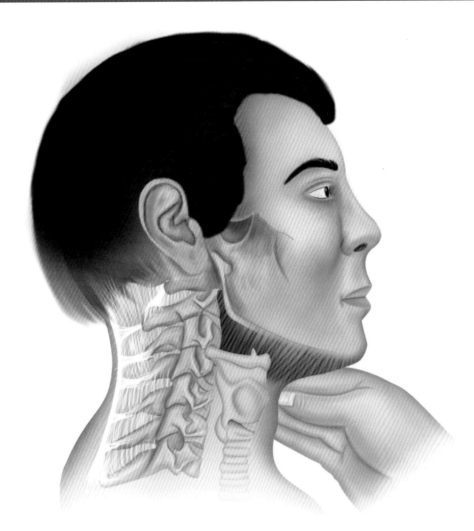

Fig. 2.4 Beginning palpation for the thyroid cartilage by starting high in the neck.

Carotid Tubercle of C6

Palpation: The carotid tubercle is found by moving laterally from the first cricoid ring (**Fig. 2.8**). Palpate the carotid tubercles one at a time. Bilateral palpation of the carotid tubercles may cause compression on both carotid arteries, causing the patient to faint (**Fig. 2.9**). Additionally, the depth of palpation necessary for this can be uncomfortable to the conscious patient. It is extremely useful to localize the C6 level when performing anterior cervical surgery.

Trachea

Palpation: Evaluate the trachea (**Fig. 2.10**) for any deviation from the midline, and note any abnormal findings.

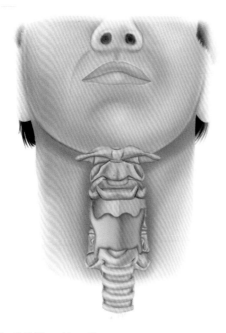

Fig. 2.5 Thyroid cartilage.

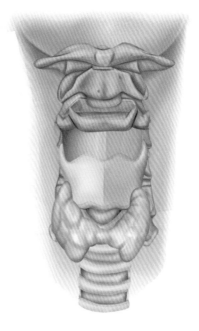

Fig. 2.6 Lateral and posterior to the thyroid cartilage is the thyroid gland.

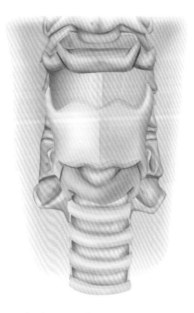

Fig. 2.7 The first cricoid ring is located just below the thyroid cartilage.

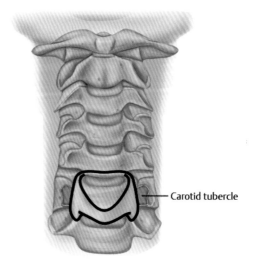

Carotid tubercle

Fig. 2.8 The carotid tubercle is found by moving horizontally and laterally from the cricoid ring.

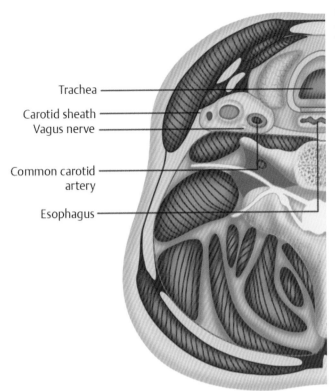

Fig. 2.9 The carotid sheath lies directly anterior to the carotid tubercle.

Trachea

Carotid sheath

Vagus nerve

Common carotid artery

Esophagus

Soft Tissue Palpation of the Anterior Cervical Spine

Carotid Pulses

Palpation: The carotid pulses are palpable just lateral to the first cricoid ring and adjacent to the carotid tubercles (**Fig. 2.11**). The pulses are palpated one at a time to avoid restricting blood flow to the brain. The pulses should be of equal strength. Also, feel for hematoma formation or thrills. Use the stethoscope at this point for auscultation.

Supraclavicular Fossa

Palpation: The supraclavicular fossa (**Fig. 2.12**) lies superior and posterior to the clavicle and lateral to the suprasternal notch. Look for any asymmetry, and palpate for any swelling or bulge.

   Findings: Enlarged lymph nodes and cervical ribs often present in the supraclavicular fossa. A large mass or asymmetry will need further investigation because of the possibility of a tumor.

Sternocleidomastoid and Mastoid Process

Palpation: Find the sternocleidomastoid muscle at its origin at the mastoid and follow it downward, palpating to its insertion on the clavicle. To find the mastoid process, start at the inion, and palpate laterally on the superior nuchal line until you feel its rounded process (**Fig. 2.13**). If the patient is able, have the person contralaterally rotate the head and ipsilaterally side bend the neck against resistance (**Fig. 2.14**). This will sometimes cause the patient's sternocleidomastoid muscle to protrude (**Fig. 2.15**). Feel for the chain of lymph nodes that runs along the medial border of the sternocleidomastoid muscle (**Fig. 2.12**).

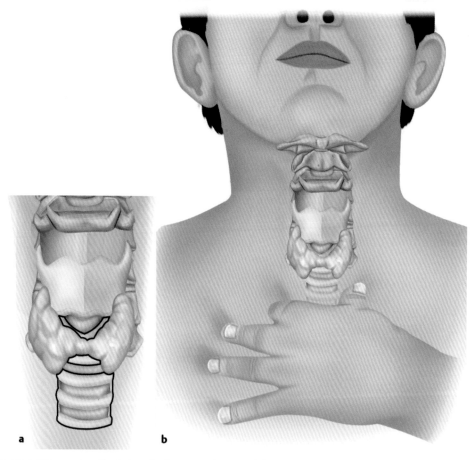

Fig. 2.10 (**a**) The trachea lies below the first cricoid ring and thyroid gland. (**b**) Palpation of the trachea.

Findings: Torticollis is the turning of the head to one side because of injury to the sterno-cleidomastoid muscle. This may result from injury to the spinal accessory nerve, swelling, and/or protective spasm of the muscle, possibly due to stretch associated with a hyperextension injury of the neck, vertebral body disease, or tonsillar infection. Enlarged lymph nodes are a possible sign of infection in the upper respiratory tract.

- Origin: sternal head—anterior surface of the manubrium; clavicular head—superior surface of the medial one-third of the clavicle
- Insertion: lateral surface of the mastoid process and lateral half of the superior nuchal line
- Nerve supply: spinal accessory nerve (cranial nerve [CN] XI) and ventral rami of C2 and C3

Parotid Gland

Begin palpating the mandible at its union (**Fig. 2.16**). Follow it posteriorly until you have reached the angle. The parotid gland lies over the angle of the mandible. If the gland is swollen, the angle of the mandible will not feel sharp.

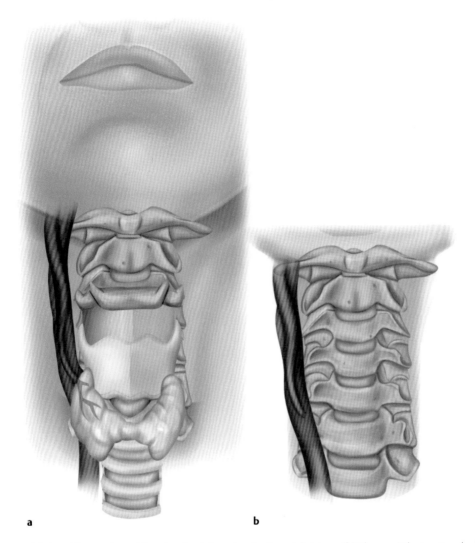

Fig. 2.11 (**a**) Carotid artery branching showing internal and external divisions. (**b**) The carotid artery is palpable just lateral to the first cricoid ring and adjacent to the carotid tubercles.

Palpation of the Posterior Cervical Spine

Following the assessment of the anterior cervical spine, the posterior aspect of the spine should be examined (**Fig. 2.17**). Bony and soft tissue palpation can be performed while the patient is seated (**Fig. 2.18a**), or while the patient is lying in the prone position on the examination table (**Fig. 2.18b**). If the patient is able to sit, the examiner should stand behind the patient. Conversely, if the patient is more comfortable lying down, the examiner should position himself or herself at the supine patient's head. Posterior bony palpation should include the occiput, the inion, the superior nuchal line posterior occipital area, spinous processes of the cervical vertebrae, and the facet joints. Soft tissue structures that should be assessed during palpation of the posterior cervical spine include the trapezius, its associated lymph nodes, and the greater occipital nerve.

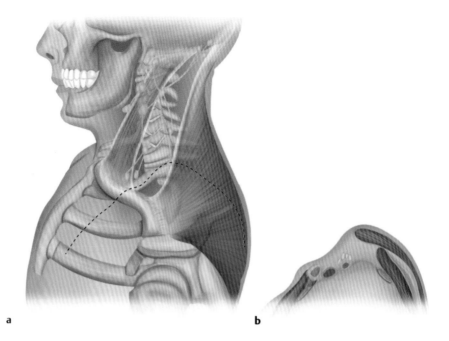

a   b

Fig. 2.12 (**a,b**) Elements of the supraclavicular fossa.

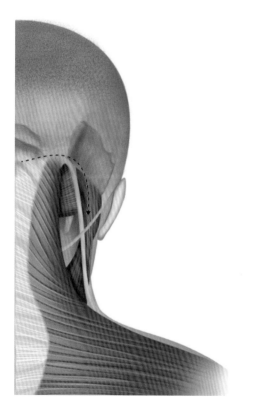

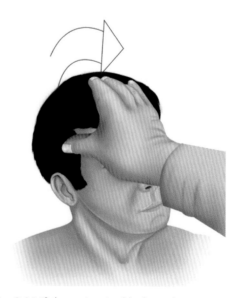

Fig. 2.13 Finding the sternocleidomastoid at its origin at the mastoid is easiest by starting at the inion and palpating laterally on the superior nuchal line until you find the rounded process.

Fig. 2.14 If the patient is able, have the person rotate the head contralaterally while side bending against resistance.

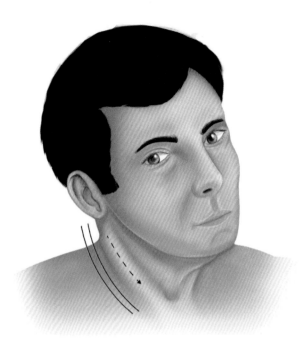

Fig. 2.15 Protrusion of the sternocleidomastoid muscle seen with contralateral rotation and ipsilateral side bending of the neck.

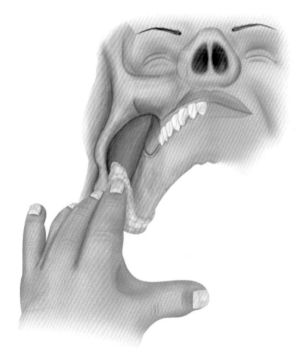

Fig. 2.16 Palpation of the parotid gland at the angle of the mandible.

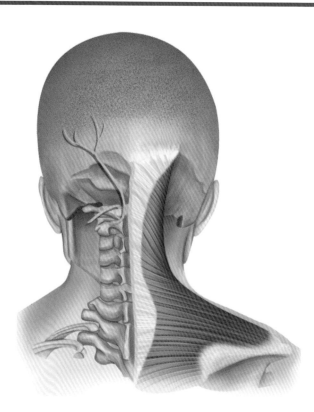

Fig. 2.17 Posterior view of the cervical spine, with bony and neural anatomy on the left (greater occipital nerve) and muscular anatomy on the right (trapezius muscle).

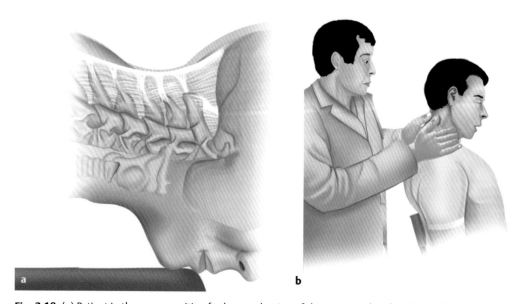

Fig. 2.18 (**a**) Patient in the prone position for bony palpation of the posterior head and neck. (**b**) Patient in the seated position for palpation of the posterior cervical spine.

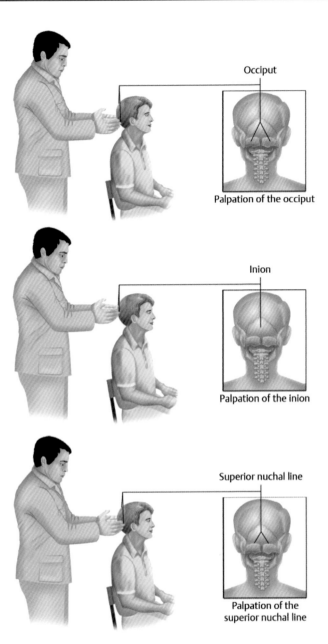

Fig. 2.19 Palpation of the occiput, superior nuchal line, and inion.

Occiput

Palpation of the occiput

Inion

Palpation of the inion

Superior nuchal line

Palpation of the superior nuchal line

Bony Tissue Palpation of the Posterior Cervical Spine

Posterior Occipital Area (Fig. 2.19)

Palpation: Standing to the left of the patient, use your right hand, thumb, and/or index finger to feel a void at the base of the skull. Move your fingers superiorly along the midline of the skull until you feel the point of a bony protuberance, the inion. As you move your fingers laterally in either direction, from the inion, you will feel a prominent bony ridge. This structure is known as the superior nuchal line. While palpating the posterior occipital area, feel for tenderness, abnormal masses, and/or bony protuberances.

Findings: For patients with odontoid (C2) fractures, sometimes tenderness is elicited with palpation of the prominent posterior C2 spinous process. Likewise, people with inflammatory

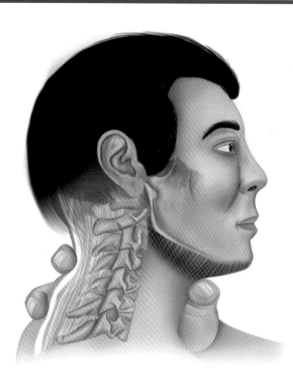

Fig. 2.20 Palpation of the spinous processes, with the thumb in the anterior midline and the fingers wrapped around the posterior aspect of the spine.

disease and/or cervicogenic pain can have pain at the insertion of their ligamentous structures on the back of the skull.

Spinous Processes

Palpation: The spinous processes are the most easily palpable bony structures in the spinal exam. Place your thumb in the anterior midline and wrap your fingers around to the posterior aspect of the spine (**Fig. 2.20**). Starting high at the base of the skull, probe with your fingers until you find the first process, C2. Continue the exam caudally and end with T1. The spinous processes should lie in line with one another. Feel for misalignments and for any curvature other than the normal lordosis of the cervical spine. Note any pain, tenderness, or swelling in the paraspinal muscles.

Facet Joints

Palpation: Begin by having the patient completely relax in the prone or seated position. Start palpation of the facet joints by moving laterally on both sides of the C2 spinous process and feel for the facet joints between the vertebrae. Continue palpating to the C7–T1 facet joint and note any tenderness elicited from the examination.

Soft Tissue Palpation of the Posterior Cervical Spine

Trapezius

Palpation: The trapezius starts bilaterally where the muscle is first located near its superior origin (**Fig. 2.21**). Find the muscle lateral and inferior to the inion, and palpate toward the acromion (**Fig. 2.22**). Feel for lymph nodes on the anterior aspect of the muscle. This chain of nodes is usually only palpable and tender from pathologic causes (infectious, tumorous, or viral). Once the acromion is reached, follow the lateral border of the muscle, palpating toward the spine of

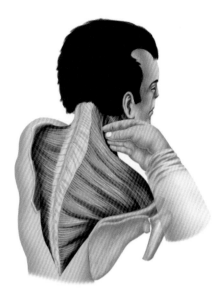

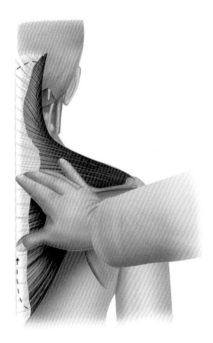

Fig. 2.21 Palpation of the trapezius muscle near its superior origin. One can feel for lymph nodes on the anterior aspect of the muscle.

Fig. 2.22 Continued palpation of the trapezius muscle at its origin on the spinous processes.

the scapula. Continue following the trapezius up along its origin on the spinal processes to the superior nuchal line.

Findings: Positive findings associated with the upper trapezius are frequently from flexion injuries as a result of whiplash. Tenderness in the area of the scapular spine insertion may also be indicative of a flexion injury of the cervical spine (**Fig. 2.23**). Tenderness here can also be related to disorders of the shoulder.

- Origin: external occipital protuberance, medial one-third of superior nuchal line, ligamentum nuchae, spinous processes from C7 to the T12
- Insertion: lateral one-third of the clavicle, acromion process, superior border and medial one-third of the spine of the scapula
- Nerve supply: spinal accessory nerve (CN XI) and ventral rami of C3 and C4

Greater Occipital Nerve

Palpation: Starting at the inion, bilaterally palpate for the greater occipital nerves. The greater occipital nerves are not normally palpable but can be sensitive.

Findings: If the greater occipital nerves are palpable/hyperaesthetic, it is probably because of inflammation as a result of a whiplash injury.

Superior Nuchal Ligament

Palpation: The superior nuchal ligament area is palpable in the midline from the inion to the C7 spinous process (**Fig. 2.24**).

Findings: Generalized tenderness may indicate a stretch from a whiplash injury. Localized tenderness is not common in cervical spondylotic disease.

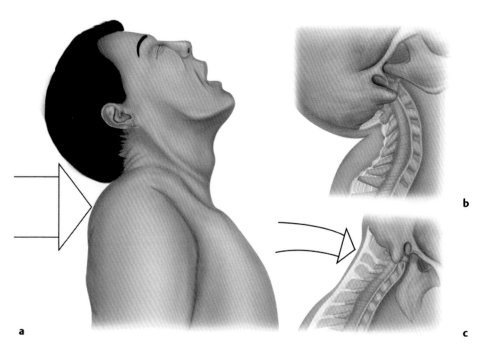

Fig. 2.23 (**a–c**) Whiplash injury can result from the depicted motions of the neck. This type of injury results in tenderness of the nuchal ligagment (**c**).

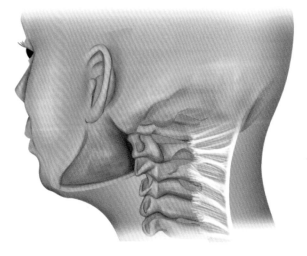

Fig. 2.24 Delineation of the superior nuchal ligament, originating on the inion, running in the midline, and attaching to the spinous processes.

■ Cervical Spine Motion Tests

Active Motions

Direct the patient to move the head in one of six directions and stop when the movement elicits pain or when the movement's range has reached its limit. The goal of the active motion exam is to determine range of motion and pattern of movement.

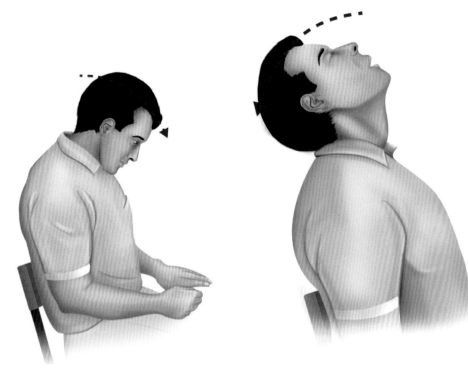

Fig. 2.25 Active neck flexion.

Fig. 2.26 Active neck extension.

Positioning: The patient should stand or sit in a normal postural position. Observe the patient's movements from behind or from the side.

Flexion

Instruct the patient to relax the jaw and bring the chin down as far as possible toward the manubrium without flexion of the thorax (**Fig. 2.25**). The patient should be able to touch the chin to the chest.

Extension

Instruct the patient to bring the head backward as far as possible without movement of the thoracic and lumbar spine (**Fig. 2.26**). As in flexion, instruct the patient to relax the jaw and leave it open to reduce tension of the platysma muscle. When the head is fully extended, the nose and forehead should be in a horizontal plane.

Left and Right Rotation

Direct the patient to turn the head as far as possible to the left and then to the right (**Fig. 2.27**). Note the limit of the patient's rotational motion. Normal rotation of the neck to one side is approximately 80 degrees. This places the chin above the shoulder. It is normal for rotational ranges to be asymmetric, but this becomes clinically important when pain is restricting motion. If one of the motions elicits pain, direct the patient to repeat the motion in flexion and then in extension. This helps load and unload the facet joints during the particular motion, with extension loading the joints.

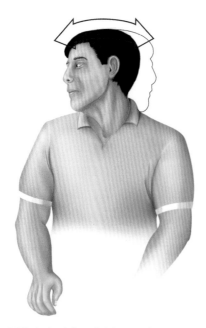

Fig. 2.27 Active left and right rotation.

Fig. 2.28 Left and right side bending.

Left and Right Side Bending

Instruct the patient to side bend the neck left and then right, without rotation, placing the ear to the shoulder (**Fig. 2.28**).

Passive Movements

When performing the passive movement examination, differences in mobility and range of motion between passive and active movements should be noted. Passive movements commonly do not elicit as much pain, so a greater range of motion can be obtained. Also, determine whether the end motion feels firm, flaccid, or rigid. Take great care to be very gentle with any patient with a history of recent trauma; do not perform passive motions until the cervical spine has been cleared for fracture or significant ligamentous injury.

Positioning: The patient should stand or sit in a normal postural position. Observe the patient's movements from behind or from the side.

Extension

To perform passive extension of the cervical spine, begin by asking the patient to open and relax the jaw. Standing by the patient's side, place your right forearm across the patient's shoulders, with your right hand on the patient's far shoulder. This steadies the body so the patient does not bend the thoracic spine with neck extension. Place the fingertips of your left hand on the patient's forehead and carefully tilt the patient's head into full neck extension (**Fig. 2.29**).

Left and Right Rotation

To test passive rotation to the left, stand behind the patient on the right side. With your left hand, cup the patient's forehead, placing your elbow on the patient's shoulder for stability. With the right hand, take hold of the back of the patient's head, and place your elbow on the

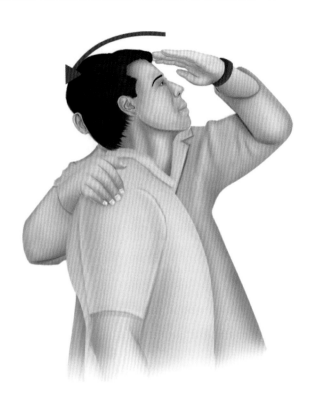

Fig. 2.29 Passive extension.

patient's right shoulder to prevent rotation of the patient's body. Slowly rotate the patient's head with both hands. Repeat the test for rotation to the right (**Fig. 2.30**).

Left and Right Side Bending

To test left side bending, place your right arm on the patient's left shoulder. Stand behind the patient. With the right arm, grasp the patient's head and rest your elbow on the posterior aspect of the patient's shoulder. Using your right arm, begin to bend the neck to the left side. Be sure to fix the body to minimize movement (**Fig. 2.31**).

■ Resisted Tests

Resistance testing of flexion, extension, rotation, and side bending is used to determine whether a lesion exists in the C1 or C2 nerve roots, which may result in muscle weakness.
   Positioning: The patient should stand or sit in a normal postural position.

Flexion

To examine resisted neck flexion, stand to the side of the patient (**Fig. 2.32**). Place one hand on the patient's forehead and the other on the posterior neck. Direct the patient to flex the neck by retracting the chin and pushing the forehead into your hand. Resist the motion.

- Primary flexor
  - Sternocleidomastoid muscle
- Secondary flexors
  - Scalenus
  - Prevertebral muscles

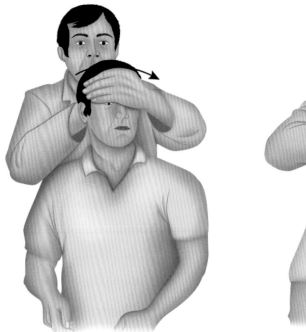

Fig. 2.30 Passive left and right rotation.

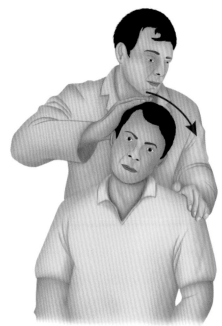

Fig. 2.31 Passive left and right side bending.

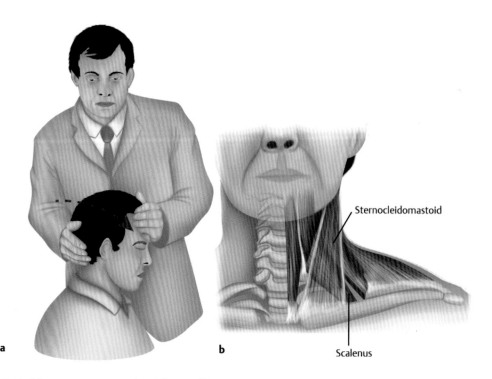

a

b

Sternocleidomastoid

Scalenus

Fig. 2.32 (**a**) Appropriate resisted neck flexion. (**b**) Musculature of neck flexion: sternocleidomastoid, scalenus, and prevertebral musculature.

Extension

To test resisted extension of the neck, stand at the patient's side, and place the palm of your hand on the patient's chest (**Fig. 2.33**). Place the elbow of your free arm on the posterior thoracic spine and that hand on the back of the head. Instruct the patient to push back with the head onto your hand. Resist the movement with an equal and opposite force.

- Primary extensors
  - Splenius
  - Semispinalis capitis
  - Trapezius
- Secondary extensors
  - Intrinsic neck muscles

Left and Right Rotation

To test resisted rotation, stand behind the patient (**Fig. 2.34**). To test rotation to the left, place your left elbow on the patient's left shoulder and place your hand on the patient's forehead. Place your right elbow on the posterior aspect of the patient's right shoulder and your right hand on the back of the patient's head. Instruct the patient to turn the head to the left, and resist the motion. Repeat the test for rotation to the right.

- Primary rotator
  - Sternocleidomastoid muscle
- Secondary rotators
  - Intrinsic neck muscles

Left and Right Side Bending

To test resisted side bending to the left, stand behind and to the left of the patient (**Fig. 2.35**). Place your left elbow on the patient's left shoulder and your palm on the patient's head, just above the ear. With the other hand, grasp the patient's right shoulder. Instruct the patient to side bend the neck to the left, and resist the motion. Repeat the test for side bending to the right.

- Primary side benders
  - Scalenus anterior, scalenus medius, and scalenus posterior
- Secondary side benders
  - Intrinsic neck muscles

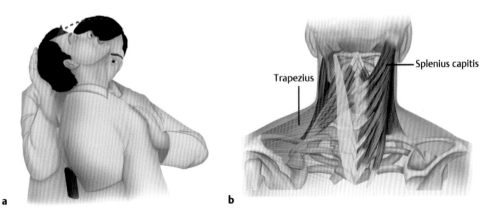

a   b

Fig. 2.33 (**a**) Appropriate resisted neck extension. (**b**) Muscles of neck extension: splenius capitis, semispinalis capitis, and trapezius.

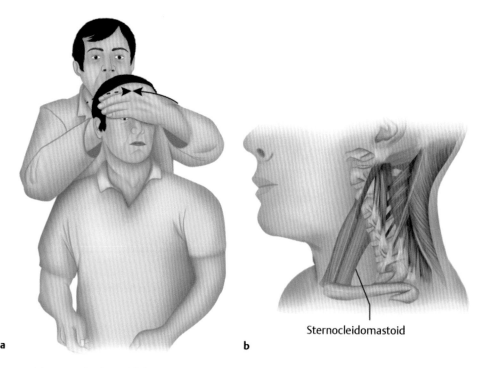

Sternocleidomastoid

Fig. 2.34 (**a**) Resisted right and left rotation. (**b**) Muscles of left and right rotation: sternocleidomastoid and intrinsic neck muscles.

Fig. 2.35 Resisted right and left side bending.

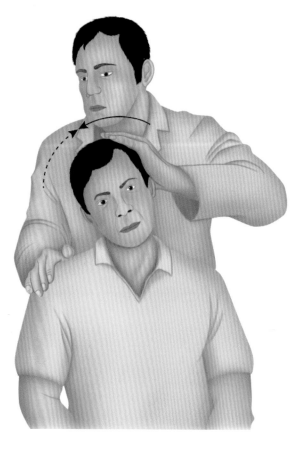

▉ Neurologic Evaluation

C2–C4

The C1–C4 nerve roots are difficult to test, and lesions to these roots usually indicate a serious condition. The diaphragm is innervated by roots C3, C4, and C5, with the majority of its nerve input from C4. A cord lesion at or above this level will result in a loss of the ability to inhale, causing significant respiratory problems, frequently with a need for mechanical ventilation.

Motor C2–C4

Resisted Bilateral Scapular Elevation

To perform bilateral scapular elevation, place the patient in a standing or seated position (**Fig. 2.36**). Stand directly behind the patient. Instruct the patient to shrug both shoulders up as high as possible. Place both hands on the patient's shoulders and attempt to push them toward the floor. This should be impossible to do when C2, C3, and C4 are intact. Weakness found in the scapular exam indicates a serious pathology. Note any differences in elevation heights or any asymmetry in strength. The spinal accessory nerve also plays a role in this motion.

- Primary elevators
  - Trapezius: CN XI
  - Levator scapulae: C3, C4, and sometimes C5

- Secondary elevators
  - Rhomboid major
  - Rhomboid minor

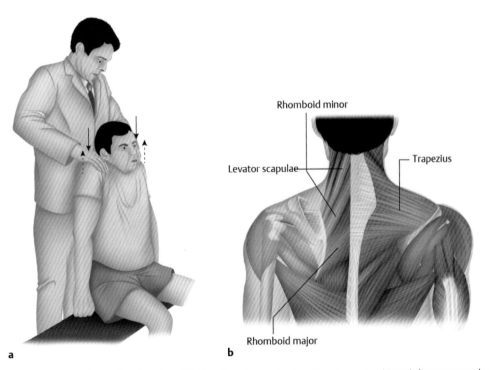

Fig. 2.36 (**a**) Resisted scapular elevation. (**b**) Muscles of scapular elevation: trapezius (CN XI), levator scapulae, rhomboid major, and rhomboid minor.

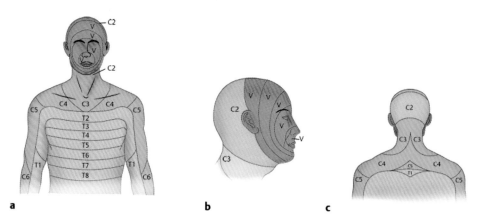

Fig. 2.37 **(a)** Sensory dermatomes of the cervical and upper thoracic spine. **(b)** Sensory dermatomes of the skull involving C2, C3, and CN V. **(c)** Sensory dermatomes of the skull and upper shoulder girdle.

Sensory C2–C4

The sensory dermatomes of C2, C3, and C4 give sensation to the back of the skull and neck (**Fig. 2.37, Fig. 2.38**). Because these roots have no significant myotome, the diagnosis of upper cervical radiculopathy relies often on these dermatomal abnormalities, which must be tested specifically with a pinwheel. The lower cervical dermatomes demonstrate a well-defined dermatomal map displayed in the figures.

C5

Motor C5

C5 is best tested by the deltoid muscle. The deltoid is innervated almost entirely by C5, whereas the biceps is innervated by both C5 and C6.

Shoulder Abduction (C5)

To perform shoulder abduction, have the patient stand or sit with the arms resting alongside the body. To test the left shoulder, stand to the left of the patient, and place your left hand on the patient's distal upper arm. Place your right hand on the hip or shoulder to stabilize the patient. Instruct the patient to push the arm into abduction, and resist the motion. Repeat the test on the right shoulder. Testing bilaterally and simultaneously provides excellent comparison between the right and left sides (**Fig. 2.39**).

- Primary abductors (**Fig. 2.40**)
  - Deltoid: axillary nerve C5, C6
  - Supraspinatus: suprascapular nerve C5, C6
- Secondary abductor
  - Serratus anterior

Shoulder Flexion (C5, C6)

To test shoulder flexion, stand behind the patient with one hand on the shoulder and the other arm wrapping around the biceps (**Fig. 2.41**). Instruct the patient to flex the elbow to 90 degrees. Then instruct the patient to flex the shoulder, bringing the arm forward. Resist the patient's movement.

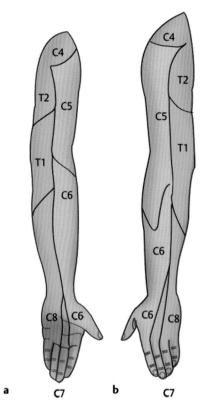

Fig. 2.38 (**a**) Ventral dermatome distribution of C4 through T2. (**b**) Dorsal dermatome distribution of C4 through T2.

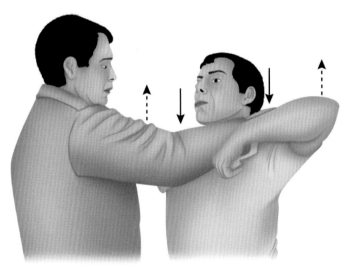

Fig. 2.39 Bilateral simultaneous shoulder abduction tests of the deltoid, supraspinatus, and serratus anterior muscles.

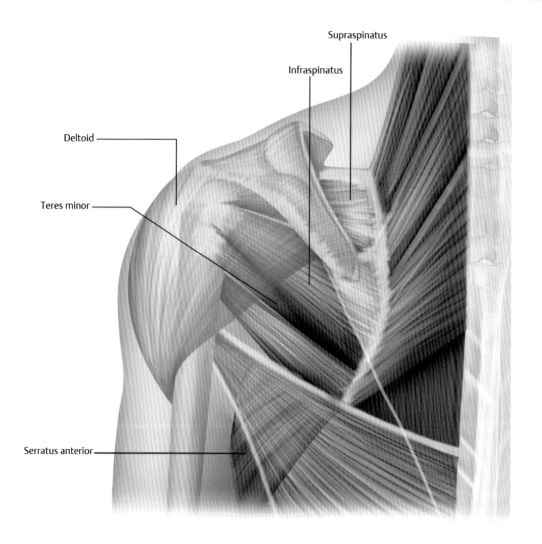

Fig. 2.40 Muscles of shoulder abduction (supraspinatus, deltoid, and serratus anterior) and muscles of external rotation of the shoulder (infraspinatus, teres minor, deltoid).

- Primary flexor
  - Deltoid: axillary nerve C5
  - Coracobrachialis: musculocutaneous nerve C5, C6
- Secondary flexors
  - Pectoralis major
  - Biceps

External Rotation of the Shoulder (C5, C6)

To test external rotation of the shoulders, have the patient stand before you with arms resting alongside the body and both elbows flexed at 90 degrees (**Fig. 2.42**). Instruct the patient to then externally rotate both hands against resistance.

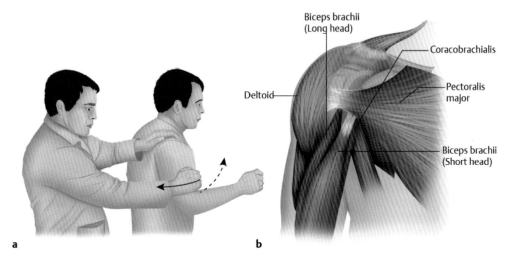

Fig. 2.41 (**a**) Shoulder flexion. (**b**) Muscles of shoulder flexion: deltoid, coracobrachialis, pectoralis major, and biceps.

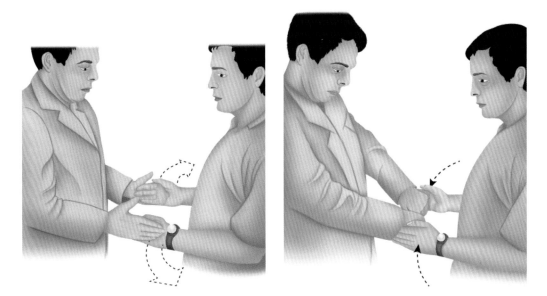

Fig. 2.42 External rotation of the shoulder.

Fig. 2.43 Internal rotation of the shoulder.

- Primary external rotators
  - Infraspinatus: suprascapular nerve C5, C6
  - Teres minor: axillary nerve C5
- Secondary external rotator
  - Deltoid

Internal Rotation of the Shoulder (C5, C6)

Test the resisted internal rotation of the shoulder in the same manner as resisted external rotation (**Fig. 2.43**). The test for internal rotation is not as accurate as those for flexion, extension, and abduction of the shoulder because of C6, C7, C8, and T1 involvement.

- Primary internal rotators (C5, C6)
  - Subscapularis: subscapular nerves C5, C6
  - Pectoralis major: C5, C6, C7, C8, T1
  - Latissimus dorsi: thoracodorsal nerve
  - Teres major: lower subscapular nerves C5, C6
- Secondary internal rotator
  - Deltoid

Elbow Flexion (C5, C6)

With the patient standing or sitting, stand in front of the patient, and place one hand on the elbow and wrap the other around the wrist. The hand on the elbow fixates the arm during the exam. The patient begins with the elbow flexed at 90 degrees and is instructed to further flex the arm. As the arm flexes, increase resistance to provide maximum resistance when the arm and forearm create an angle of approximately 45 degrees. Care should be taken to ensure full supination of the wrist to test the C5 myotome (**Fig. 2.44, Fig. 2.45**). Patients with C5 weakness will inadvertently cheat by pronating the wrist and use the C6 innervated muscle to resist.

- Primary flexors
  - Brachialis: musculocutaneous nerves C5, C6
  - Biceps: musculocutaneous nerve C5, C6
- Secondary flexors
  - Brachioradialis
  - Supinator

Sensory C5

C5 is tested by its sensory contribution to the axillary nerve. It supplies sensation to the lateral aspect of the upper arm (**Fig. 2.38**).

Biceps Reflex: C5

Instruct the patient to sit or stand with the left forearm flexed and relaxed at an angle of 90 degrees. Face the patient, standing to the person's left side. The patient's forearm rests over your left forearm. Grasp the patient's left elbow with your left hand, placing your thumb over the biceps tendon. Strike your thumb over the tendon with the reflex hammer, watching for contraction of the biceps muscle (**Fig. 2.46**).

C6

Motor C6

Motor testing of the C6 nerve root is difficult because the testable muscles of C6 are also partially innervated by other nerve roots. Because the wrist extensors have a larger C6 contribution, they can be used for testing along with the biceps (**Fig. 2.47**).

Elbow Flexion (C5, C6)

See C5 level motor testing for instructions.

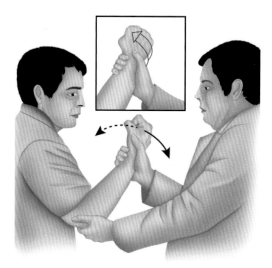

Fig. 2.44 Elbow flexion. Care should be taken to resist pronation (movement shown in box) in an attempt to keep the test to that of pure biceps function (C5).

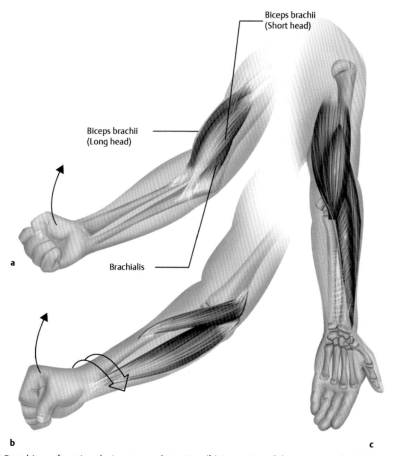

Fig. 2.45 (**a**) Pure biceps function during strength testing. (**b**) Pronation of the wrist, results in the pronator assisting forearm musculature during elbow flexion. This leads to C6 innervation during a test to assess C5 innervation. (**c**) Attachment and alignment of the biceps and forearm musculature while the wrist and forearm are supinated.

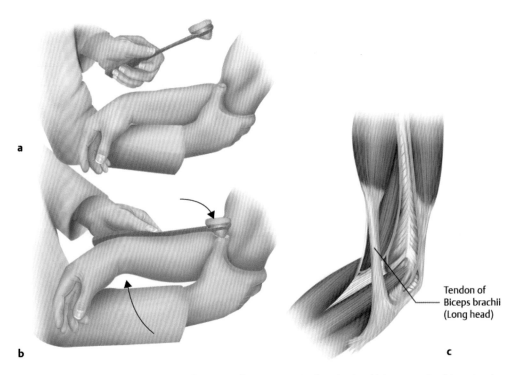

a

b

c

Tendon of
Biceps brachii
(Long head)

Fig. 2.46 (**a**) Position for the biceps reflex test. The examiner's thumb should be over the bicep tendon. (**b**) Biceps reflex is a slight flexing of the elbow. (**c**) Biceps with tendon attachment.

Fig. 2.47 (**a**) Resisted wrist flexion. (**b**) Muscles of wrist flexion.

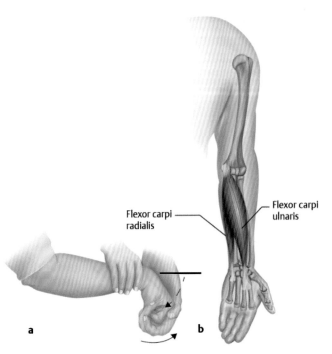

Flexor carpi
radialis

Flexor carpi
ulnaris

a

b

Wrist Extension (C6)

Have the patient stand with the arms at the sides and relaxed. Position yourself to the left of the patient. Grasp the patient's elbow at the proximal forearm. Place your free hand on the dorsal aspect of the patient's hand. Instruct the patient to extend the wrist against resistance (**Fig. 2.48**). Alternatively, have the patient extend the wrist and attempt to force the wrist into flexion (**Fig. 2.49**). Unbreakable strength is 5/5.

- Primary extensors
  - Extensor carpi radialis longus: radial nerves C5, C6
  - Extensor carpi radialis brevis: radial nerves C5, C6
  - Extensor carpi ulnaris: radial nerve C6

Sensory C6

C6 is tested by its sensory contribution to the musculocutaneous nerve. It supplies sensation to the lateral forearm, thumb, index finger, and one-half of the middle finger (**Fig. 2.38**).

Brachioradialis Reflex: C6

Instruct the patient to sit or stand with the forearm flexed and relaxed at an angle of 90 degrees. Face the patient, standing to the person's right. To test the patient's left brachioradialis reflex, rest the patient's forearm on your right forearm. Grasp the patient's arm with your right hand over the triceps. Using the reflex hammer, strike the brachioradialis tendon at the musculotendinous junction in the midportion of the radius to elicit a jerk (**Fig. 2.50**). Repeat the test on the right arm.

C7

Motor C7

Motor function of C7 is tested by the strength of the triceps and the flexors of the wrist. For triceps testing, have the patient attempt to push you away as you hold the arm in elbow flexed position. With the wrist flexed, attempt to extend the wrist.

Shoulder Adduction

To test for shoulder adduction, have the patient sit or stand with the arms hanging alongside the body. Place a hand either on the hip or on the shoulder for body stabilization (**Fig. 2.51**). Grasp the elbow with your other hand. Instruct the patient to hold the arm close to the body as you forcefully try to abduct the arm.

- Primary adductors
  - Pectoralis major: C5, C6, C7, C8, T1
  - Latissimus dorsi: thoracodorsal nerves C6, C7, C8
- Secondary adductors
  - Teres major
  - Deltoid

Elbow Extension

With the patient standing or sitting, stand in front of the patient. Place one hand on the elbow, and grasp the patient's wrist with the other hand (**Fig. 2.52**). The hand on the elbow fixes the arm during the exam. With the elbow fully flexed, instruct the patient to extend the arm. As the

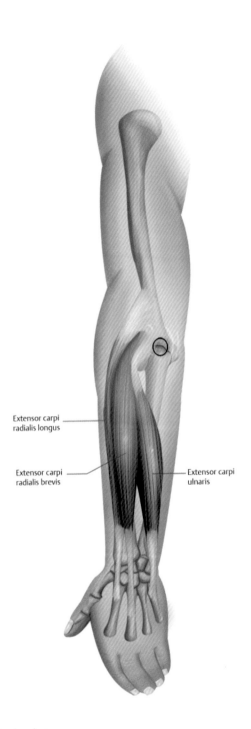

Extensor carpi
radialis longus

Extensor carpi
radialis brevis

Extensor carpi
ulnaris

Fig. 2.48 Muscles of wrist extension.

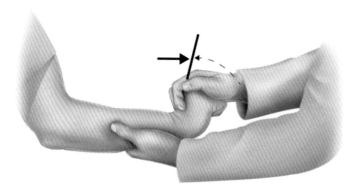

Fig. 2.49 Alternate wrist extension test. The patient extends the wrist, and the examiner attempts to force the hand into flexion.

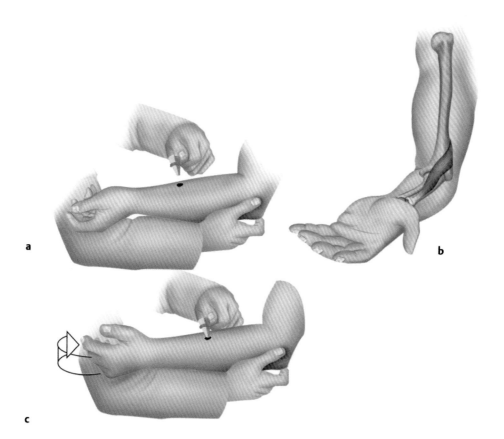

Fig. 2.50 (**a**) Brachioradialis reflex target for reflex hammer. (**b**) Brachioradialis. (**c**) Reflex arc with wrist extension.

arm extends, increase resistance to provide maximum resistance when the arm and forearm create an angle of approximately 60 degrees.

- Primary extensor
  - Triceps: radial nerve C7
- Secondary extensor
  - Anconeus

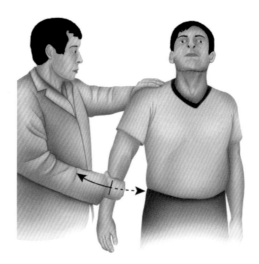

Fig. 2.51 Shoulder adduction.

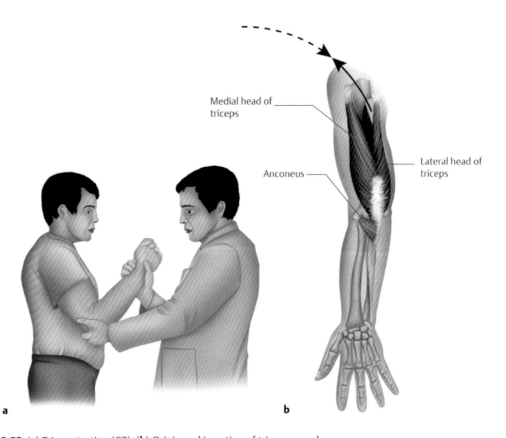

Medial head of triceps

Anconeus

Lateral head of triceps

a

b

Fig. 2.52 (**a**) Triceps testing (C7). (**b**) Origin and insertion of triceps muscle.

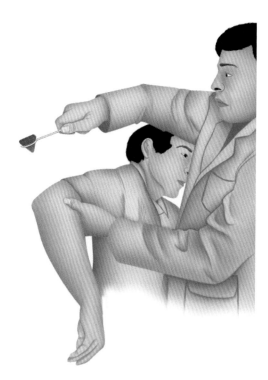

Fig. 2.53 Testing triceps reflex.

Wrist Flexion

To test wrist flexion, instruct the patient to make a fist and grasp the hand from the palmar side (**Fig. 2.47**). Hold the underside of the patient's wrist with the other hand for support. Instruct the patient to flex the wrist while you attempt to pull it into extension.
* Primary flexors
  - Flexor carpi radialis: median nerve C7
  - Flexor carpi ulnaris: ulnar nerve C8

Sensory C7

C7 most commonly provides sensation to the middle finger, although sensation is sometimes supplied by C6 and C8 (**Fig. 2.38**).

Triceps Reflex: C7

To test the triceps reflex, stand in front of the patient and grasp the inner aspect of the arm. Instruct the patient to fully relax the arm. To elicit a jerk, tap the triceps tendon with the reflex hammer just proximal to the olecranon where the tendon crosses the olecranon fossa (**Fig. 2.53**).

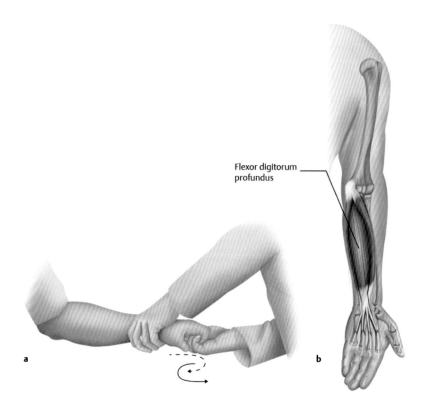

Flexor digitorum profundus

a

b

Fig. 2.54 (**a**) Testing finger flexion. (**b**) Muscles of finger flexion.

C8

Motor C8

Motor function of C8 is best tested by finger flexion and thumb adduction.

Finger Flexion C8

To test finger flexion, instruct the patient to make a fist. Curl your fingers under the patient's fingers and try to extend them. Grasp and secure the arm and wrist of the patient with your free hand (**Fig. 2.54**).

- Primary flexors
    - Flexor digitorum profundus: ulnar nerve and anterior interosseous branch of median nerves C8, T1
    - Flexor digitorum superficialis: median nerves C7, C8, T1

Adduction of the Thumb

To test thumb adduction, the patient's palm faces upward. Stabilize the wrist by holding the ulnar side of the wrist and hand. Take hold of the thumb in an abducted position and instruct the patient to adduct the thumb against resistance (**Fig. 2.55**).

- Primary adductor
    - Adductor pollicis: ulnar nerve C8

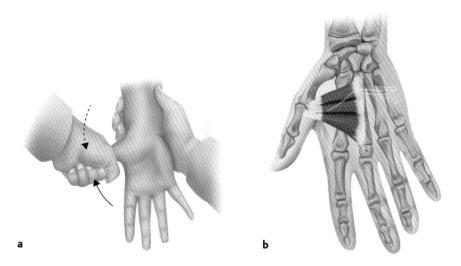

Fig. 2.55 (**a**) Testing thumb adduction. (**b**) Muscle of thumb adduction: adductor pollicis.

Sensory C8

C8 provides sensation to the ulnar side of the distal forearm, the ring finger, and the little finger (**Fig. 2.38**).

T1

Motor T1

Motor function of T1 is best tested by finger abduction and adduction.

Little Finger Adduction

To test finger adduction, instruct the patient to abduct the little finger. Grasp the patient's wrist for support with the index finger of your other hand, and hook the patient's abducted little finger (**Fig. 2.56**). Further instruct the patient to adduct the little finger against the resistance.

- Primary adductor
  - Palmar interossei: ulnar nerves C8, T1

Finger Abduction

To test finger abduction, hold the patient's wrist for support. Instruct the patient to extend and spread the fingers. Attempt to adduct the fingers in pairs. First, adduct the index and middle fingers, then the middle and ring fingers, and finally the ring and little fingers.

- Primary abductors (**Fig. 2.57**)
  - Dorsal interossei: ulnar nerves C8, T1 (**Fig. 2.58**)
  - Abductor digiti minimi: ulnar nerves C8, T1 (**Fig. 2.59**)

Sensory T1

T1 is tested through its sensory contribution to the medial brachial cutaneous nerve. It supplies sensation to the medial side of the distal upper arm and proximal forearm.

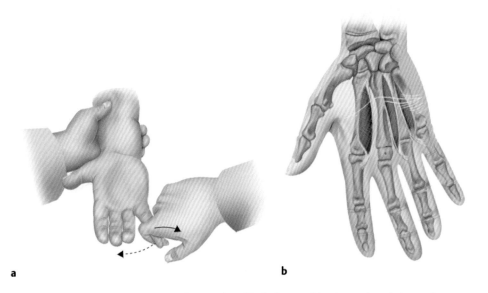

Fig. 2.56 (**a**) Testing little finger adduction. (**b**) Muscles of little finger adduction: palmar interossei.

Fig. 2.57 Testing finger abduction.

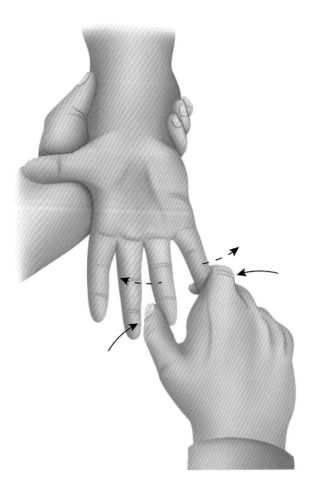

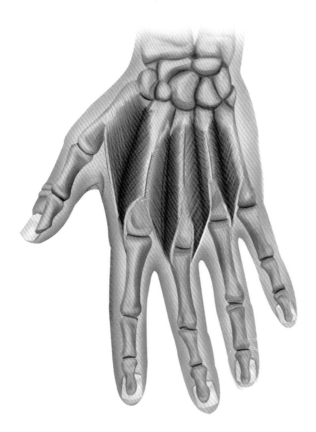

Fig. 2.58 Muscles of finger abduction: dorsal interossei.

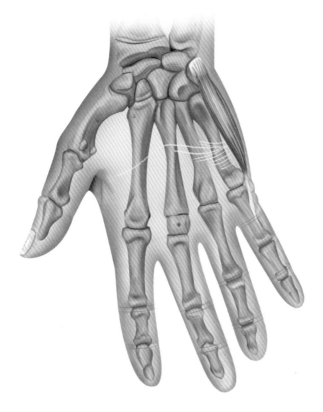

Fig. 2.59 Abductor digiti minimi.

■ Special Tests

Provocative Maneuvers

Foramina Compression Test (Left and Right) (Modified Spurling's Maneuver)

To test for foramina compression, stand behind the seated patient. Place a hand on the side of the patient's head above the ear. The other hand rests on the patient's shoulder for support. Move the head into a slight rotation and side bend to one side, while at the same time extending the patient's neck (**Fig. 2.60**). Once the head is in the correct position, add a brief axial pressure to the head. A positive test results in a root compression, indicating inadequate space in the intervertebral foramina.

Lhermitte's Test (or Phenomenon)

This phenomenon is often reported by patients as shocks or weakness in their arms and/or legs whenever they bend their head forward. To test this, ask the patient to flex the head forward, and determine if symptoms occur in a shooting fashion down the arms and/or legs (**Fig. 2.61**). This usually is caused by anterior compressive lesions, which are made worse by flexion and are a sign of myelopathy.

Axial Separation (Distraction) Test

Use this test to help determine appropriate treatment and the effects of neck traction. To perform the axial separation test, stand to the left of the seated patient. Hold the patient's head

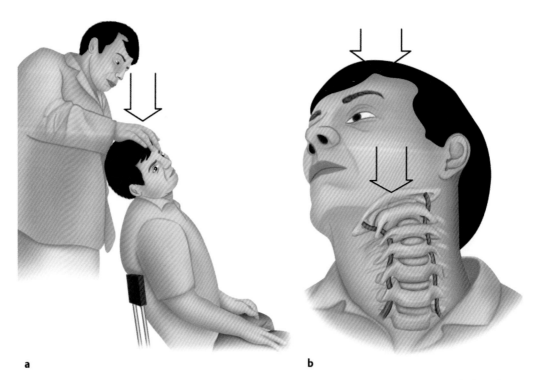

a   b

Fig. 2.60 (**a**) Modified Spurling's maneuver. (**b**) Mechanism of foraminal compression with modified Spurling's maneuver.

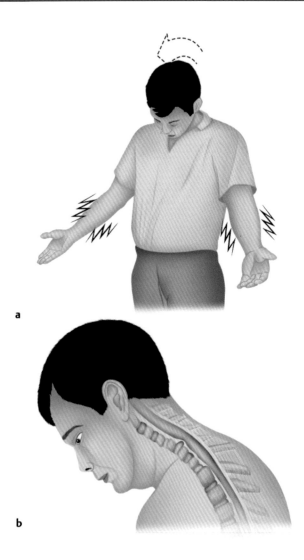

Fig. 2.61 (a) Lhermitte's test (or phenomenon): flexion of the neck, causing sensations into the arms from spinal cord compression. (**b**) Mechanism of spinal cord compression in Lhermitte's phenomenon.

a

b

with the right hand under the occiput and the left hand beneath the mandible. Perform a distraction of the head. This is performed in slight flexion and extension and in a neutral position (**Fig. 2.62**).

Valsalva Test

Valsalva test is used to detect space-occupying lesions in the spinal canal (**Fig. 2.63**). To perform this test, instruct the patient to hold the breath and bear down, as when lifting weights improperly or straining to empty the bowels. If this action produces or increases preexisting pain or other symptomatology, the test is positive. Note in which dermatomes the patient feels the pain; this could be indicative of the cord level of the lesion. Positive Valsalva tests can be caused by herniated disks or tumors.

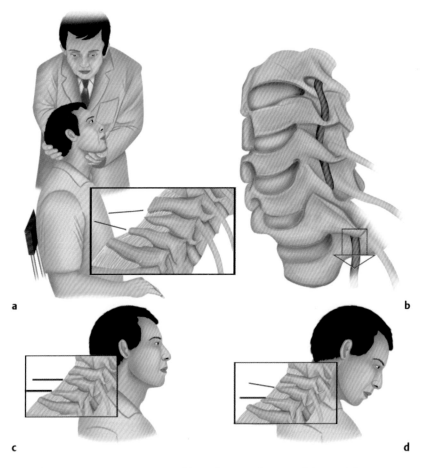

Fig. 2.62 (**a**) Axial separation (distraction) test. (**b**) Mechanism of action of the axial distraction test opening. (**c**) Effect of extension in the axial distraction test. (**d**) Effect of flexion in the axial distraction test.

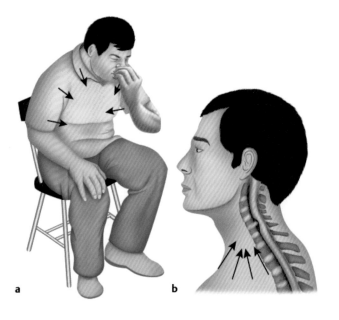

Fig. 2.63 (**a**) Valsalva test. (**b**) Mechanism of intra-abdominal pressure leads to heightened irritation of the spinal cord or other symptomatology with Valsalva test. Increase in spinal cord with preexistent pathology.

Examination of the Blood Vessels

Modified DeKleyn and Nieuwenhuyse Test

To perform the modified DeKleyn and Nieuwenhuyse test, have the patient rest in a supine position with the head over the edge of the exam table. Support the head with both hands. Perform the following passive movements for 2 minutes each, returning the head to a neutral postural position for at least 1 minute between motions (**Fig. 2.64**): extension; rotation (left and right); extension with rotation and side bend to the same side (**Fig. 2.65**); flexion with rotation to one side and side bend to the opposite side. Stop the examination if a symptom is reproduced and remains for 15 seconds. The test is positive if a motion performed during the examination elicits a new symptom that persists or the same symptom as the patient's complaint (**Fig. 2.66**). Once a position is found positive, the exam ends without performance of the other positions.

If the patient complains of dizziness, vestibular dysfunction must be ruled out before considering vertebrobasilar syndrome. Dizziness elicited during the combined movement of extension with rotation is considered by some to be pathognomonic of vertebrobasilar syndrome.

Adson's Test

Use the Adson's test to determine compression of the subclavian artery (**Fig. 2.67**). To perform this test, locate the radial pulse on the wrist with the patient sitting or standing. Continue to feel the pulse as you abduct, extend, and externally rotate the patient's arm. Once the arm is in the proper position, instruct the patient to take a deep breath, hold it, and rotate the head toward the tested arm. The test is positive if the pulse is reduced or lost. A positive test indicates compromise or compression of the subclavian artery. This can occur as the result of the existence of a cervical rib or tightened scalenus anticus and scalenus medius muscles.

Vertebral Artery Motion Test

Use the vertebral artery motion test to determine if vertebral artery symptoms are elicited by movements that stress the arteries (**Fig. 2.68**). To perform the vertebral artery motion exam, instruct the patient to stand with the legs shoulder width apart. Stand in front of the patient,

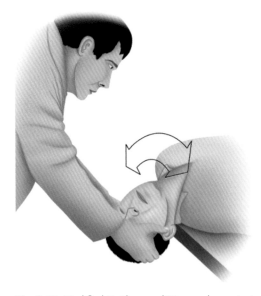

Fig. 2.64 Modified DeKleyn and Nieuwenhuyse test.

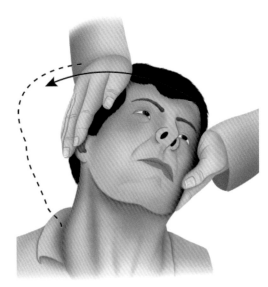

Fig. 2.65 Rotation and side bending during modified DeKleyn and Nieuwenhuyse test.

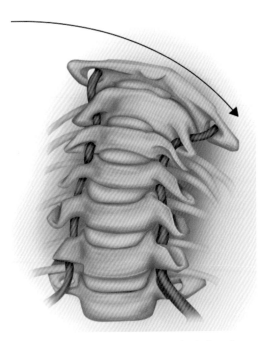

Fig. 2.66 Mechanism of arterial compression during rotation and side-bending maneuver.

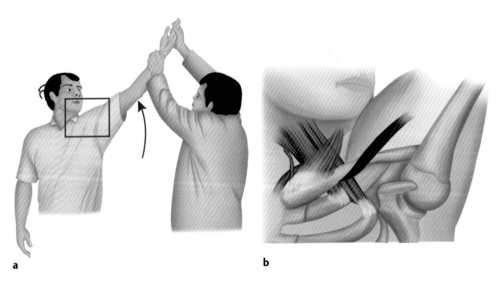

a b

Fig. 2.67 (a) Adson's test. (b) Mechanism of arterial compression during Adson's test.

and place both hands on the shoulders to keep the patient's body from moving. Instruct the patient to rapidly turn the head from side to side for 10 seconds or until symptoms are reproduced. If the exam produces symptoms, check to see if the pupils are symmetric. Asymmetric pupils after the vertebral artery motion test may indicate reduced blood flow through one of the vertebral arteries.

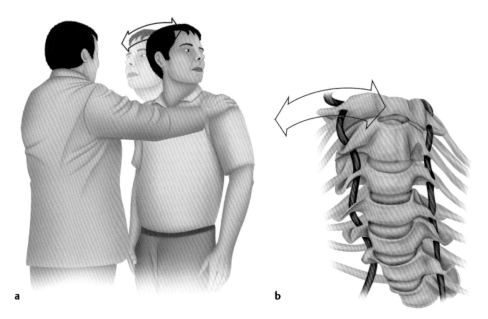

a   b

Fig. 2.68 (**a**) Vertebral artery motion test. (**b**) Mechanism of production of vertebral artery symptoms due to stress of vertebral arteries during motion test.

Cervical Rib Exam

To perform the cervical rib exam, palpate the radial pulse, and apply traction to the patient's arm (**Fig. 2.69**). If the pulse is reduced or lost, it may suggest a cervical rib. Evidence of ischemia in one hand and a murmur of the subclavian artery may also indicate an obstruction caused by a cervical rib. Bilateral symptoms of ischemia are suggestive of other pathologic conditions such as Raynaud's disease.

Upper Motor Neuron Evaluation

Hoffmann's Test

Hoffmann's test is used to determine an upper motor neuron lesion above T1. To perform the Hoffmann's test, instruct the patient to completely relax the hand. Flick the nail of the middle finger. If the muscles of the hand and thumb flex, the patient has a positive Hoffmann's sign. This indicates that a lesion originates in the central nervous system and is not a radiculopathy or a peripheral nerve lesion (**Fig. 2.70**).

Crossed/Inverted Radial Reflexes

Another sign of cord irritation/myelopathy, spasticity, or disinhibition, this pathologic reflex occurs when the reflex arc spreads beyond the normal expected response. For example, when percussing the biceps tendon with a hammer, both a biceps reflex and a wrist extensor reflex are elicited (crossed radial reflex) (**Fig. 2.71**). When the brachioradialis is struck, both a wrist extensor and finger flexor responses are elicited (inverted radial reflex) (**Fig. 2.72**). Both findings should prompt investigation for cord compression.

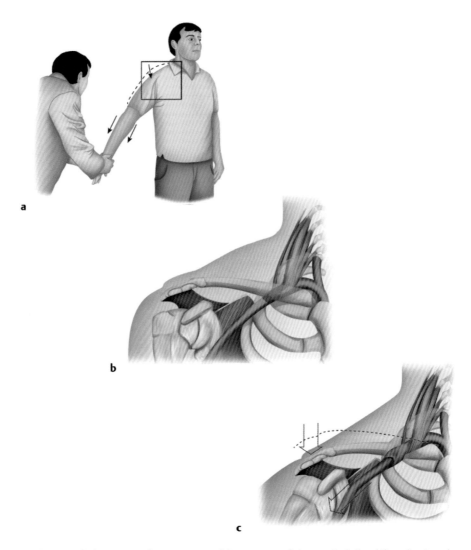

Fig. 2.69 (**a**) Cervical rib exam applying traction. (**b**) Anatomy of the cervical rib while palpating the radial pulse. Reduction or loss of radial pulse. (**c**) Compression of the subclavian artery with the cervical pulse is suggestive of a cervical rib.

Static/Dynamic Romberg's Test

To perform the static Romberg's test, have the patient stand with the hands outstretched and palms up with the arms at 90 degrees of flexion (**Fig. 2.73**). Then have the patient close the eyes. If the patient loses balance or falls backward, or if the arms rise slowly to above parallel, it is a sign of proprioceptive deficit either from central (possibly cerebellar) dysfunction or from myelopathy.

For the dynamic Romberg's test (also known as heel–toe walking), instruct the patient to walk in a straight line, heel to toe (**Fig. 2.74**). Difficulty doing so is often a sign of proprioceptive deficit, as above.

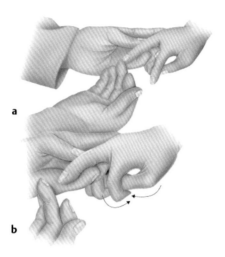

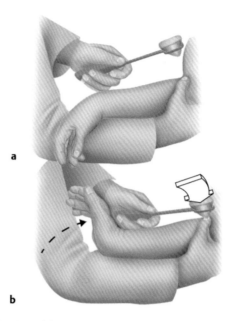

Fig. 2.70 (a) Hoffmann's test. **(b)** Positive Hoffmann's test with finger and thumb flexion after flicking the middle fingernail.

Fig. 2.71 (a) Testing for biceps reflex. **(b)** Elicitation of crossed radial reflex with wrist extension upon percussion of biceps reflex.

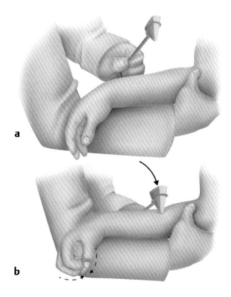

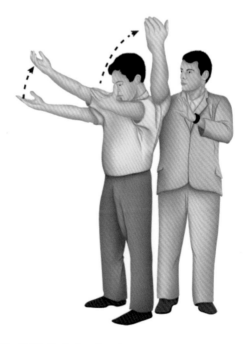

Fig. 2.72 (a) Testing for brachioradialis reflex. **(b)** Elicitation of inverted radial reflex with finger flexion upon percussion of the brachioradialis.

Fig. 2.73 Static Romberg's test.

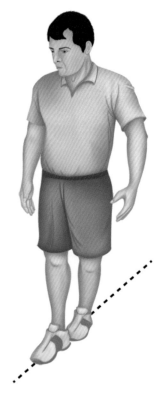

Fig. 2.74 Dynamic Romberg's test (also known as heel–toe walking).

Babinski's Sign

To perform the Babinski's test, take the patient's foot with one hand. Using the handle of the reflex hammer or a sharp object, stroke the bottom of the foot. Starting at the heel, pull the handle of the reflex hammer along the lateral plantar surface of the foot.

When the tuberosity of the fifth metatarsal is reached, turn and stroke in a medial direction toward the tuberosity of the big toe (**Fig. 2.75**). Proper initiation of the reflex may require a strong and forceful stroke. The test is positive if the big toe extends. A positive Babinski's sign indicates an upper motor neuron lesion. It should be included as a test to rule out cervical and/or thoracic myelopathy in all spinal examinations.

Clonus (Fig. 2.76)

To detect clonus, have the patient in the seated position and ask them to relax. Take the patient's foot with both hands while it is in the neutral position, and forcibly position the foot into dorsiflexion. If this elicits downward beats of the foot into an equinus position more than once or twice, it is generally abnormal and a sign of spinal cord irritation. This test should be repeated on the other foot and the results should be compared.

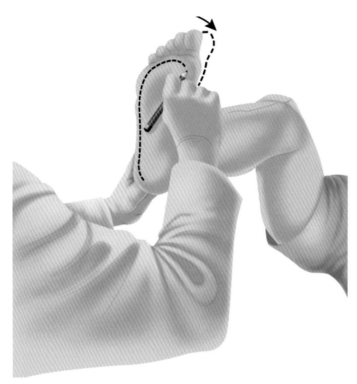

Fig. 2.75 Babinski's sign (S2, S3). The test is positive if the big toe extends, indicating an upper motor neuron lesion. Normally the toes curl downward with this maneuver.

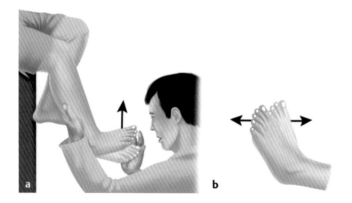

Fig. 2.76 (**a**) Test for clonus in the seated position (**b**) positive clonus response.

Chapter 3

Physical Examination of the Thoracic Spine

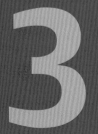

3 Physical Examination of the Thoracic Spine

Examination of the thoracic spine differs from that of the cervical and lumbar sections. Thoracic nerve roots, with the exception of T1, do not innervate the musculature of the extremities. Thoracic nerve root localization and testing therefore occur through palpation, movement, and sensory examination.

■ Visual Examination

General Impression

The examination begins as the patient enters the room. First notice if the patient is distressed. Is the patient leaning to one side, and is the patient able to walk? If so, is the person's gait normal? As in the cervical examination, ask the patient to disrobe, and stay in the room to observe. Note if the patient is limited in any motion, and note the extent of any pain elicited. Once the patient is undressed, look for signs of trauma, blisters, scars, discoloration, redness, contusions, lumps, bumps, hairy patches, café au lait spots, fat pads, and other marks.

Assessing Alignment

During visual evaluation of the thoracic and lumbar spine, it is important to pay close attention to the alignment and curvatures of the spine in the sagittal (lateral) and coronal (frontal) planes. While performing this exam, ask the patient to stand in their "normal posture."

To visualize the sagittal plane, stand to the left or the right of the patient (**Fig. 3.1**). If the patient exhibits truncal inclinations that deviate from "normative posture" or an abnormal anterior (forward) or posterior (backward) rotation of the pelvis (pelvic tilt), a detailed evaluation of the entire spine should be performed.

To visualize the coronal plane, stand directly in front of the patient, then walk around the patient to view the back of the spine. While evaluating the spine in the coronal plane, it is important to pay close attention to the concave and convex curvatures of the spine (**Fig. 3.2**), the height of the patient's shoulders, and degree of pelvic obliquity. Any abnormal observations or discrepancies should be documented, and a detailed scoliosis evaluation should be performed.

■ Palpation

During the physical evaluation, the patient should be gowned, and their back should be facing you. Begin by feeling the general surface temperature over the thoracic spine using the backs of the hands. Compare one side with the other. Note any areas of sweating or pain, and use caution when palpating these areas.

Spinous Processes

To palpate the spinous processes of the thoracic spine, begin by finding C7 or T1 (**Fig. 3.3**). These are the most prominent of the spinous processes and can easily be found by running a finger

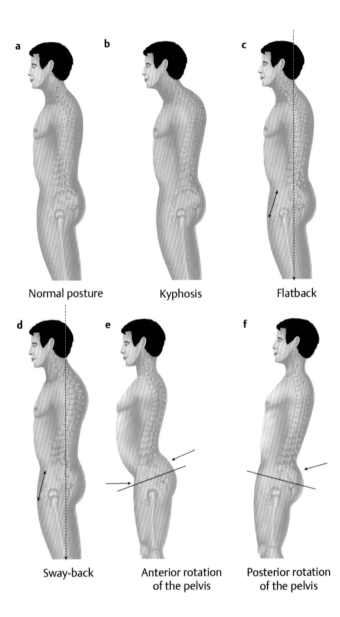

Fig. 3.1 Examples of common postural abnormalities and pelvic rotations in the sagittal plane. (**a**) Normal posture. (**b**) Kyphosis. (**c**) Flatback. (**d**) Sway-back. (**e**) Anterior rotation of the pelvis. (**f**) Posterior rotation of the pelvis.

a   b   c

Normal posture   Kyphosis   Flatback

d   e   f

Sway-back   Anterior rotation of the pelvis   Posterior rotation of the pelvis

down the midline of the flexed neck. Place the thumb of each hand on the spinous processes and begin to palpate, in a caudal direction, until you have traveled past the ribs (**Fig. 3.4**). Note any misalignments, curvature, lumps, pain, tenderness, and/or swelling.

Facet Joints

To palpate the facet joints of the thoracic spine, instruct the patient to relax completely. Again begin by finding C7 or T1. Move your fingers laterally from the spinous processes, feeling for the facet joints between the vertebrae (**Fig. 3.5, Fig. 3.6a**). Continue palpating caudally to the end of the thoracic spine. Note if tenderness is elicited by the examination. Palpate the ribs, the costovertebral articulations, and along the intercostal bundles, looking for sensitivity or pain elicitation (**Fig. 3.6b**).

63

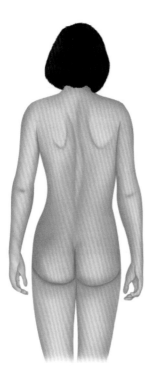

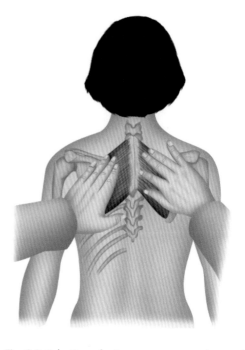

Fig. 3.3 Palpation of spinous processes and paraspinal musculature of the thoracic spine.

Fig. 3.2 Posterior view of a patient with scoliosis. Notice the right scapular elevation and spinal curvature. The patient should be told to fully extend the knees and have the arms at the sides when being visually inspected.

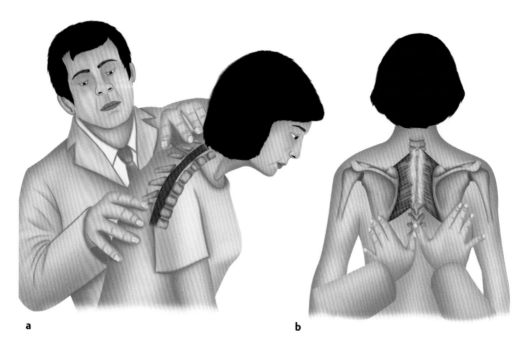

a

b

Fig. 3.4 (**a**) Palpation of the upper thoracic spine. (**b**) Palpation of the thoracic spine, including the facet joints.

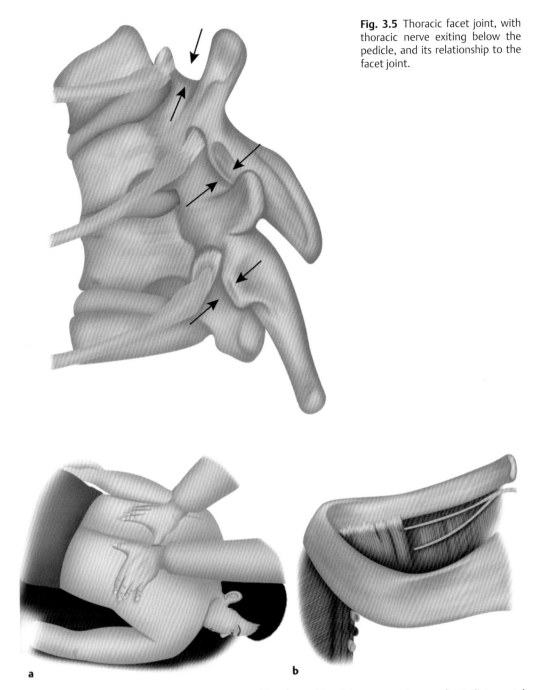

Fig. 3.5 Thoracic facet joint, with thoracic nerve exiting below the pedicle, and its relationship to the facet joint.

Fig. 3.6 (a) Palpation of the thoracic facet joints. (b) Relationship of the nerve, artery, and vein (intercostal bundle) below the rib.

■ Percussion

Instruct the patient to bend over and flex the back. Lightly percuss the back, beginning with the base of the neck and moving down toward the sacrum (**Fig. 3.7a**). Marked pain elicited during percussion is sometimes found in tuberculous and other infections. It also suggests the possible presence of a compression fracture and is a useful way to follow the healing of these fractures (**Fig. 3.7b**).

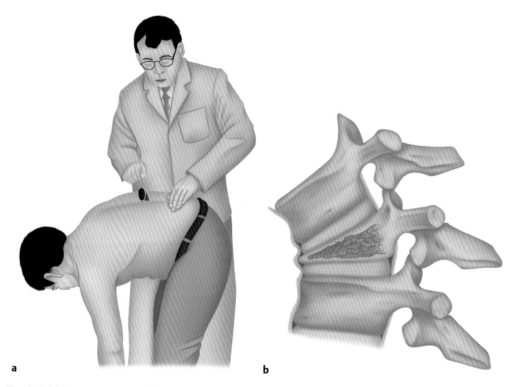

a   b

Fig. 3.7 (**a**) Percussion across thoracic vertebrae with a reflex hammer. This can help to identify an area of tenderness or a compression fracture. (**b**) Example of a thoracic compression fracture with wedging of the vertebral body and acute kyphosis.

■ Movements

Active Movements

Bending Forward

Ask the patient to bend over and touch the toes without bending the knees. Take note of flexibility, fluidity, and restriction of movement. Do this from both a standing (**Fig. 3.8a**) and a sitting (**Fig. 3.8b**) position.

Bending Backward

To examine thoracic extension, palpate the spinous processes of T12 and L1. Instruct the patient to fully extend the spine by bending backward (**Fig. 3.9**). Place one hand on the back of the patient to detect the point at which the spinal extension moves into the lumbar vertebrae.

Side Bending

To test active side bending, instruct the patient to cross the arms, resting the hands on the opposite shoulders (**Fig. 3.10**). Ask the patient to side bend to the left and then to the right. The crossing point of the arms will form an imaginary axis of rotation. Note any pain or limitations in movement.

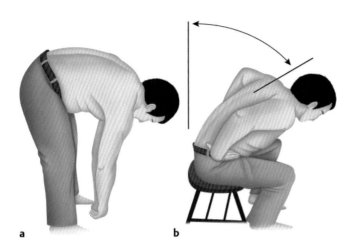

Fig. 3.8 (**a**) Forward bending from a standing position. (**b**) Forward bending from a sitting position.

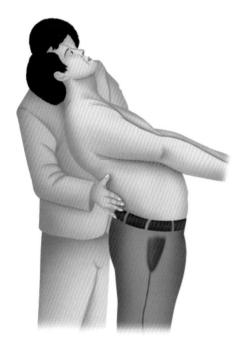

Fig. 3.9 Thoracic extension.

Trunk Rotation

Thoracic trunk rotation occurs with the patient seated with arms crossed and hands resting on opposite shoulders (**Fig. 3.11**). A wedge or block is placed under the patient's buttock on the side being tested.

The elevation of the buttock will lock the lumbar spine in contralateral side bending and ipsilateral rotation. Instruct the patient to rotate as far as possible toward the side where the block was placed. The cervical spine is not rotated. Note any pain or limitations in movement.

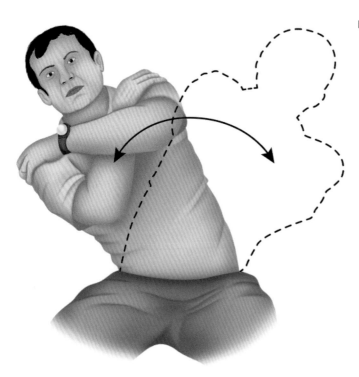

Fig. 3.10 Thoracic side bending.

Passive Movements

Passive tests are employed when full range of motion is not achieved during active testing. Passive tests of flexion are not performed because of possible aggravation if a disk protrusion exists.

When testing passive movements, take note of the end feel, range of motion, and any pain elicited. Do not push beyond the painful limits.

Rotation

To perform passive rotation, instruct the patient to sit on the examination table with the buttock of the side being tested resting on a wedge or block. The patient's arms are crossed, and the hands are rested on the opposite shoulders. The patient's feet are placed flat on the floor. Once the patient is in position, stand in front, straddle the patient's legs, and place both hands on the shoulders. Finally, rotate the patient in the direction to be tested (**Fig. 3.12**).

Resisted Movements

Rotation

To perform resisted rotation, instruct the patient to sit with arms crossed and hands placed on opposite shoulders. Stand in front of the patient. To test rotation to the left, place your right arm on the patient's right shoulder. Your left hand is placed on the back of the patient's right shoulder. Ask the patient to rotate to the left against the resisting force. Repeat for rotation to the right (**Fig. 3.13**).

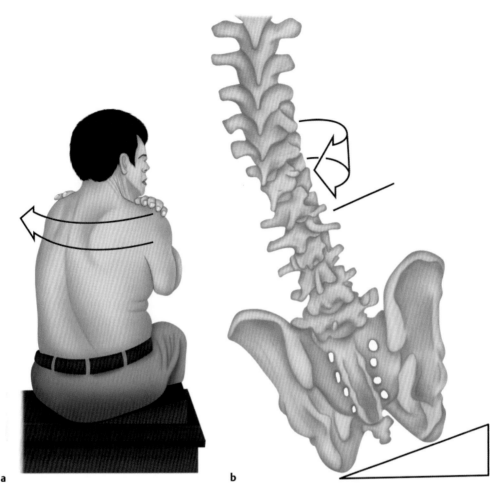

Fig. 3.11 (**a**) Trunk rotation. This is performed with a wedge or block under the patient's buttock on the side being tested. (**b**) Example of how the block under the side to which the spine is rotated locks the lumbar spine rotation.

Flexion

To perform resisted flexion, stand to the side of the patient. Place one hand on the back over the thoracic–lumbar junction and the other on the chest over the manubrium (**Fig. 3.14**). Instruct the patient to flex as you resist. Note any weakness or pain.

Side Bend

To test resisted side bending, sit next to the seated patient. Wrap one arm around the patient's back, and place the other hand on the patient's shoulder (**Fig. 3.15**). Sit close to the patient, and place the lateral side of your pelvis against the patient's pelvis to lock it into place. Instruct the patient to side bend away from you, and resist the motion. Note any weakness or pain.

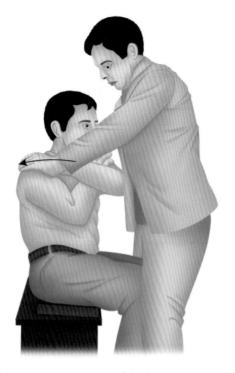

Fig. 3.12 Passive rotation of the thoracic spine.

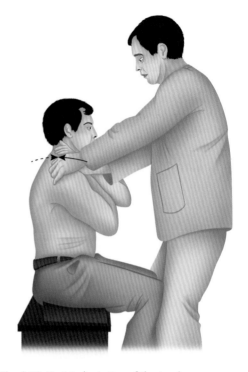

Fig. 3.13 Resisted rotation of the trunk.

Fig. 3.14 Resisted flexion of the trunk.

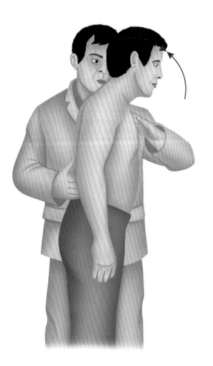

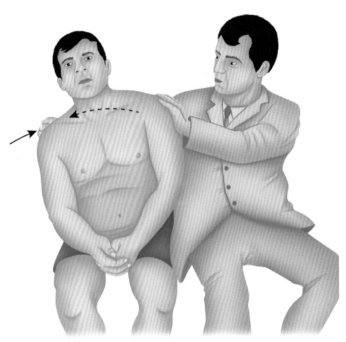

Fig. 3.15 Resisted side bending.

■ Neurologic Evaluation

Motor

Thoracic roots other than T1 innervate the intercostal, abdominal, and paraspinal muscles. It is impossible to localize root levels by testing these muscles. Localization of thoracic nerve root injury is therefore best tested by sensory evaluation (**Fig. 3.16, Fig. 3.17**).

Sensory

Significant overlap exists in sensory innervation of the thoracic region; any particular area of skin is innervated by three different nerve roots.

Three major landmarks for sensory levels exist in the thoracic region. These are the nipple line, which represents T5; the umbilicus, which represents T10; and the inguinal region, which represents the lower thoracic and upper lumbar levels (**Fig. 3.18**).

Reflex

Abdominal Reflexes and Beevor's Sign

The abdomen is segmented into four quadrants by horizontal and vertical lines passing through the umbilicus. Abdominal musculature above the umbilicus is innervated by root levels T7–T10. Musculature below the umbilicus is innervated by levels T10–L1.

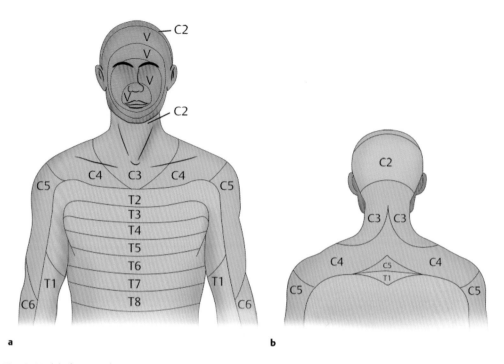

Fig. 3.16 (**a**) Thoracic dermatomes anteriorly. (**b**) Upper posterior dermatomal distribution of C2–T1.

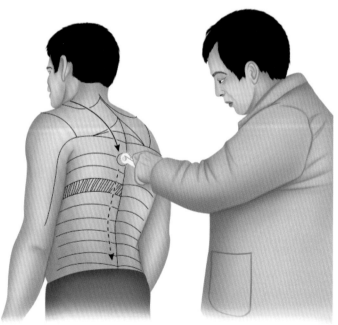

Fig. 3.17 Sensory dermatomal testing with a pinwheel down the thoracic dermatomaes.

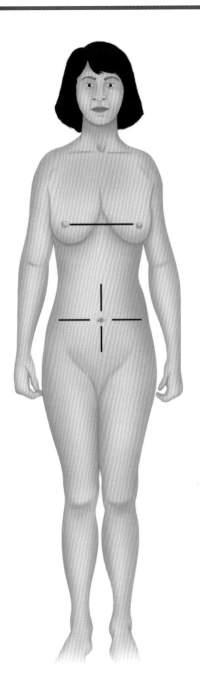

Fig. 3.18 Landmarks for sensory levels in the thoracic region: the nipple line representing T5, the umbilicus representing T10, and the inguinal region representing lower thoracic and upper lumbar regions.

To test the abdominal reflexes, instruct the patient to undress above the waist and lie supine on the examination table, totally relaxed. Individually stroke each quadrant of the abdomen lightly. The umbilicus normally migrates toward the quadrant being stroked. Diminished movement may indicate an upper motor neuron lesion. An asymmetric loss of the reflex may indicate a lower motor neuron lesion (**Fig. 3.19**).

Next, have the patient do a sit-up. If the umbilicus moves upward during the sit-up, it implies a lesion at T10 or below. If downward motion occurs, the potential lesion is at T10 or above (**Fig. 3.20**). Asymmetric movement here is the Beevor's sign (the test is the Beevor's test).

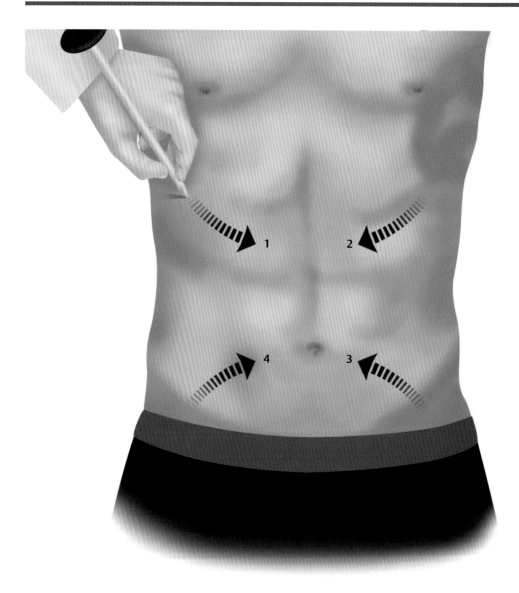

Fig. 3.19 Abdominal reflex test.

Rib Expansion Test

Stand facing the patient, then place your open hands on the patient's chest/rib cage and feel for equal and significant rib cage expansion during inhalation (**Fig. 3.21**). Absent or poor expansion may be indicative of ankylosing spondylitis or a motor lesion affecting the diaphragm (C3, C4, C5, or above).

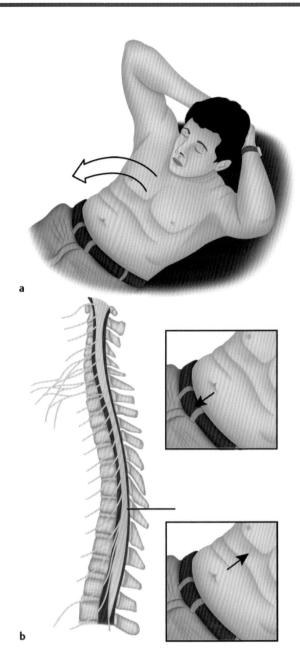

Fig. 3.20 (**a**) Abdominal musculature above the umbilicus is innervated by T7–T10. Musculature below the umbilicus from T10–L1. If the umbilicus moves up when the patient performs a sit-up, the lesion is at T10 or below. If downward motion occurs, the lesion is at T10 or above. (**b**) Neurology of the Beevor's test. The level of lesion is designated by motion of the umbilicus when performing a sit-up.

Spinal Dysraphism

During development of the spine from notochordal tissue in the embryo, abnormalities can occur that affect the spinal cord, nerve roots, and spinal column. Abnormalities such as these are referred to as spinal dysraphism and include spina bifida, diastematomyelia (split cord), and tethered cord. The presence of such abnormalities can be suggested by hair patches and sinuses on the skin overlying the spine and cord. These should be specifically investigated (**Fig. 3.22**).

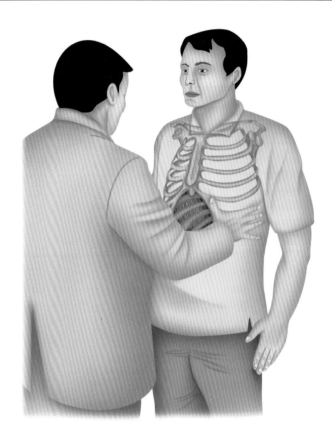

Fig. 3.21 Rib expansion test. Absence or poor expansion of the ribs on inhalation may be indicative of ankylosing spondylitis or a motor lesion affecting the diaphragm (C3–C4, C4–C5, or above).

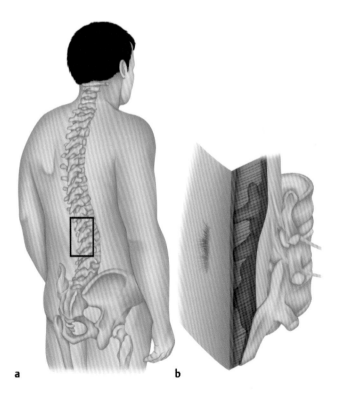

Fig. 3.22 (**a**) Common area of spinal dysraphism. (**b**) Spinal dysraphism is suggested by hair patches, which may be indicative of spina bifida, a split spinal cord, or a tethered cord. Inspection of the skin should be performed for hair patches or sinuses.

a   b

■ Deformity Evaluation

Physical Evaluation

The thoracic spine should naturally have some degree of forward curvature, called kyphosis. An excessive forward curvature of the thoracic spine results in a deformity known as hyper kyphosis. This deformity can significantly impact a patient's physical function and quality of life. To evaluate the degree of kyphosis, the spine should be viewed from the side (**Fig. 3.1**). Excessive rounding of the upper back and shoulders is a strong indicator that the angle of kyphosis has exceeded normal values. To further evaluate thoracic kyphosis, ask the patient to bend forward at the waist until their chest is parallel to the ground (**Fig. 3.23**). Once the patient is in the correct position, look for rounding of the thoracic spine. In the clinic, radiographs and tools like the goniometer should be used to measure the angle of kyphosis. It should be noted that there can be a disparity between the patient's clinical presentation and radiographic findings. Assessing the flexibility of the thoracic kyphosis will help determine the intervention needed to correct the forward curvature. This can be done by having the patient lie in a prone position on an exam table (**Fig. 3.24**).

In the coronal plane, the spine should have a straight and vertical alignment. Abnormal lateral curvature of the thoracic spine is caused by the inclination (scoliosis) of the thoracic vertebral bodies. Scoliosis evaluation should begin by holding a weighted string to the C7 spinous process to create a plumb line (**Fig. 3.25a**). This line should pass through the center of the gluteal fold. Deviation to the right or left is measured in centimeters and recorded as a coronal decompensation in either direction. The Adam's forward bend test should be conducted to determine if a

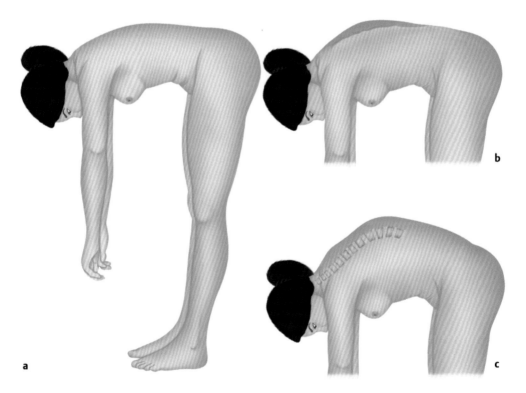

Fig. 3.23 (**a**) Estimation of sagittal curvature and kyphotic angulation grossly by having the patient bend forward and evaluating the thoracic kyphosis. (**b**) Thoracic kyphosis evaluation. (**c**) Thoracic kyphosis with apex approximately at T8.

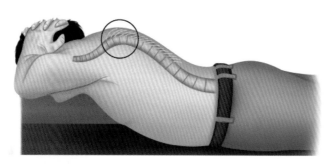

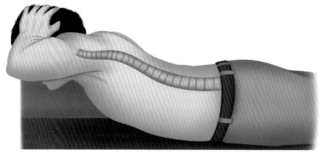

Fig. 3.24 Evaluating flexibility of thoracic kyphosis by patient extension. This can help distinguish between postural kyphosis and fixed structural kyphosis.

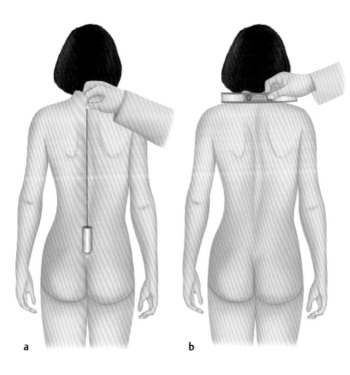

a   b

Fig. 3.25 (**a**) Plumb line dropped from the C7 (vertebra prominens) should fall in the gluteal cleft for perfect spinal balance. The number of centimeters to the right or left the plumb line falls from the C7 vertebra is used as a measure of coronal imbalance. (**b**) Evaluation of shoulder heights. The level should be placed across the shoulder at the top of the scapula. Notice the right shoulder elevation in this patient.

thoracic or lumbar prominence exists, implying spinal rotation (**Fig. 3.26**). The prominence is measured by a scoliometer (**Fig. 3.27**), giving an angular reading, or by measuring the height of the prominence directly and recorded in centimeters (**Fig. 3.28**). Measuring and comparing a patient's shoulder height (right vs. left) (**Fig. 3.25b**) and examining the orientation of the pelvis will provide further insight into the nature of the deformity and strategies for treatment (if necessary). To gauge the flexibility of the scoliotic deformity, perform a three-point bending test (**Fig. 3.29**). The flexibility of the deformity can be further evaluated by unweighting the curve (**Fig. 3.30**).

During deformity evaluation of the thoracic spine, it is important to keep in mind that malalignment found in this region can either result as a compensatory mechanism for deformities in the cervical or lumbar spine, or drive deformities in the other regions. Full-length anteroposterior (AP) and lateral scoliosis X-rays or a full body biplanar X-ray should be ordered to further evaluate the degree and nature of the deformity, to assess global alignment of the spine, and to create an effective surgical plan (if needed).

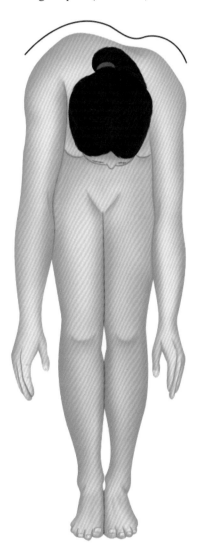

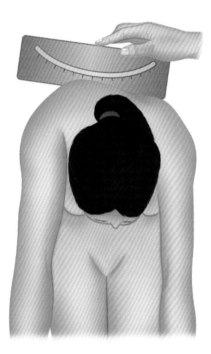

Fig. 3.27 Using a scoliometer to measure the angle of prominence. This is reported in degrees comparing the elevated side to the nonelevated side.

Fig. 3.26 Adam's forward-bending maneuver. The spinal rib hump can be clearly estimated by viewing the patient's back from superior/inferior and comparing the elevated side (convexity) to the lower side. It is usually reported as number of centimeters of elevation.

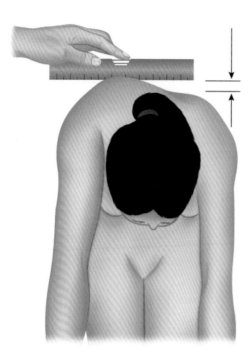

Fig. 3.28 Using a level to estimate the centimeters of rib hump elevation.

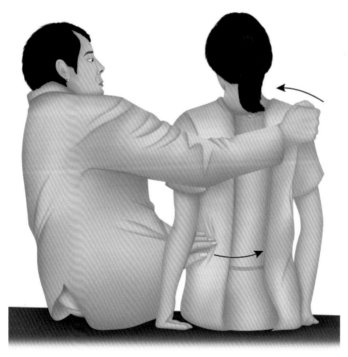

Fig. 3.29 Measurement of spinal flexibility with three-point bending to estimate the correctability of the scoliotic curvature.

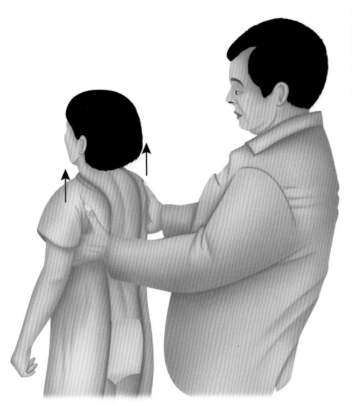

Fig. 3.30 Measurement of curve correctability. The spine is unweighted by lifting the patient from under the axillae. This is the equivalent of a traction maneuver to see how much correction is obtained with the traction.

Medical History

While conducting a deformity evaluation, it is imperative to obtain a full medical history from the patient with specific details relating to skeletal maturity and growth (especially in adolescent idiopathic scoliosis). The risk for deformity progression is directly related to skeletal growth velocity. Maximal skeletal growth occurs 6 months prior to and 6 months after menarche in a female. In males, it is more difficult to pinpoint maximal skeletal growth velocity. As a result, growth velocity is judged indirectly by pubic hair development and growth measures. Developing a detailed understanding of the patient's medical history will help determine the underlying cause of deformity, which plays a crucial role in planning and navigating an effective treatment plan.

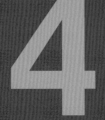

4 Physical Examination of the Lumbosacral Spine

The nerve roots of the lumbar and sacral spine, like those of the cervical spine, innervate musculature in the extremities. Through testing of the sensory and motor function of the lower extremities, you will be able to localize a cord or root injury.

■ Inspection

When the patient enters the room, notice if he or she is distressed. Is the patient leaning to one side? Is the patient able to walk, and if so, is the gait normal? Pay attention to the pelvis, taking note of any tilt. Imaginary lines through both the anterosuperior and posterosuperior iliac spines should be in a horizontal plane with the floor. As in the cervical and thoracic examination, ask the patient to disrobe, and stay in the room to observe. Note if the patient is limited in any motion, and note the extent of any pain. Once the patient is undressed, look for signs of trauma, blisters, scars, discoloration, redness, contusions, lumps, bumps, fat pads, and other marks. Hairy patches or café au lait spots imply spinal dysraphism, and neurofibromatosis specifically. Next, instruct the patient to stand with normal posture. Look at the spine from the side, and assess the lumbar curvature with the normal lordosis. If possible, instruct the patient to bend over and flex the spine, and look for a lateral curvature, or scoliosis. If a lateral curvature is seen, ask the patient to sit, and reexamine the lumbar spine. Note if the lateral curvature persists.

■ Palpation

Posterior Lumbar, Sacral, and Coccygeal Spine

To palpate the posterior lumbar, sacral, and coccygeal spine, sit on a stool behind the standing patient. Place your thumbs on the midline of the patient's back at the level of the iliac crest. This should be the junction between L4 and L5, called the interspace (**Fig. 4.1**). From the interspace, palpate superiorly and inferiorly the spinous processes of the lumbar and sacral vertebrae. Absence of spinous processes may indicate spina bifida.

The coccyx is palpable through a rectal examination that is performed in combination with the examination for sphincter tone (**Fig. 4.2**) and sacral root defects (**Fig. 4.2b**), if necessary. This is done with the patient in a lateral decubitus position (**Fig. 4.2a**) to reduce discomfort to the patient and is usually performed at the end of the examination.

Paraspinal Muscles

Instruct the patient to stand and extend the neck. Palpate the paraspinal muscles on each side of the midline simultaneously (**Fig. 4.3**). Deep massage and kneading are used to detect tenderness, spasm, muscular defect, and asymmetries.

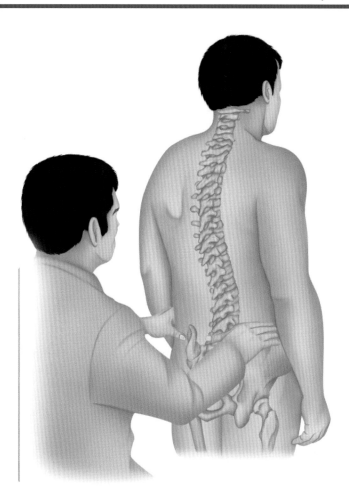

Fig. 4.1 Palpation of the lumbar spine.

Anterior Lumbar, Sacral, and Coccygeal Spine

To perform palpation of the anterior lower spine, instruct the patient to lie supine on the exam table with knees bent and muscles completely relaxed (**Fig. 4.4**).

The vertebral bodies and disks of L4, L5, and S1 can be palpated just below the umbilicus. To do this, ask the patient to relax. Push firmly into the abdomen, and feel for the vertebral bodies. The L5–S1 articulation is the most prominent bony feature found. Hyperextension of the lumbar spine makes palpation easier. This examination can be extremely difficult if not impossible on the obese patient.

■ Movements

Active Movements

Forward Bending

To test forward bending, ask the patient to bend over and touch the toes without bending the knees (**Fig. 4.5**). Take note of fluidity and any areas of restricted movement.

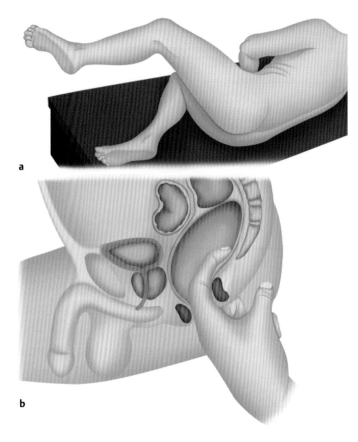

Fig. 4.2 (a) Palpation of the coccyx is performed most comfortably with the patient in the lateral decubitus position. **(b)** Coccygeal palpation through rectal examination can be performed in combination with the examination for sphincter tone and sacral root defects.

a

b

Backward Bending

To examine lumbar extension, place a hand on the patient's lower back over the posterior superior iliac spine. Instruct the patient to fully extend the spine by bending backward (**Fig. 4.6**). Take note of the fluidity and range of lumbar extension.

Side Bending

To test active side bending, instruct the patient to cross the arms and rest the hands on the opposite shoulders. Ask the patient to side bend to the left and then to the right (**Fig. 4.7**). The crossing point of the arms makes an imaginary axis of rotation. Place a hand on the iliac crest of the patient for stabilization. Note any pain and limitations in movement.

Trunk Rotation

Lumbar trunk rotation occurs with the patient standing, arms crossed and hands resting on opposite shoulders. Make sure that the patient keeps the chin directed perpendicular to the shoulders so that the cervical spine is not rotated.

Place a hand on the iliac crest of the side the patient is going to rotate away from. Place the other hand on the patient's opposite shoulder. The patient should rotate in each direction separately (**Fig. 4.8**).

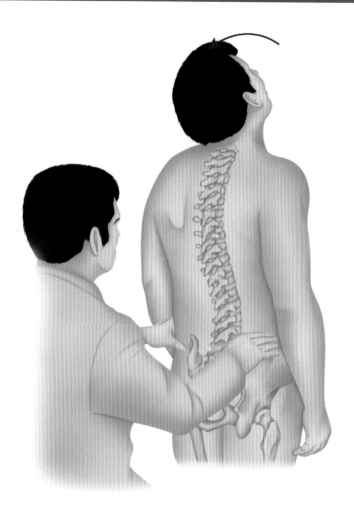

Fig. 4.3 Palpation of the paraspinal muscles and the posterosuperior iliac spine.

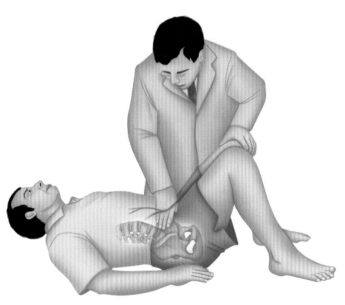

Fig. 4.4 Palpation of the anterior lumbar spine can be performed with the patient supine, knees bent, and abdominal muscles completely relaxed.

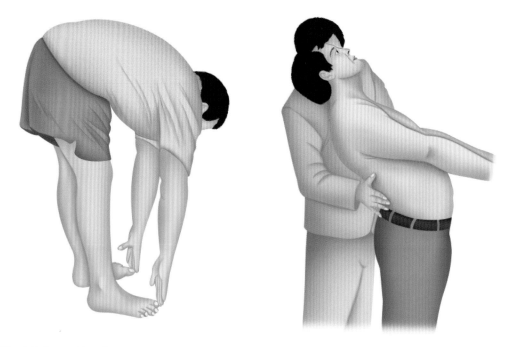

Fig. 4.5 Forward bending.

Fig. 4.6 Lumbar extension.

Fig. 4.7 Lumbar side bending.

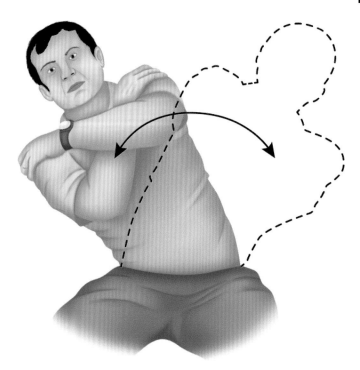

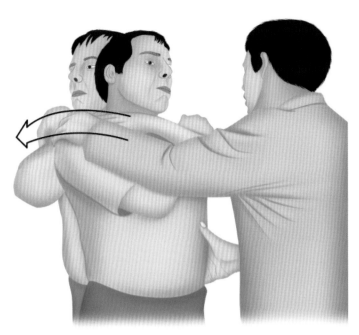

Fig. 4.8 Trunk rotation.

Passive Movements

Passive tests are employed when full range of motion is not achieved during active testing. Passive tests of flexion are not performed because of possible aggravation if a disk protrusion exists. When testing passive movements, take note of the end feel, range of motion, and any pain elicited.

Rotation

To perform passive rotation, instruct the patient to stand with their arms crossed and hands rested on opposite shoulders. Once the patient is in position, stand behind the patient and place one hand on the iliac crest and the other hand on the patient's shoulder. Finally, rotate the patient in the tested direction (**Fig. 4.9**).

Resisted Movements

Rotation

To perform resisted rotation, instruct the patient to sit with arms crossed and hands resting on opposite shoulders (**Fig. 4.10**). Stand in front of the patient. To test rotation to the left, place your left hand on the patient's left arm and your right hand on the back of the patient's left shoulder. Then ask the patient to rotate to the left against the resisting force.

Flexion

To perform resisted flexion, stand to the side of the patient. Place one hand on the patient's back over the posterosuperior iliac spine and the other hand on the chest over the manubrium (**Fig. 4.11**). Instruct the patient to flex as you resist. Note any weakness or pain.

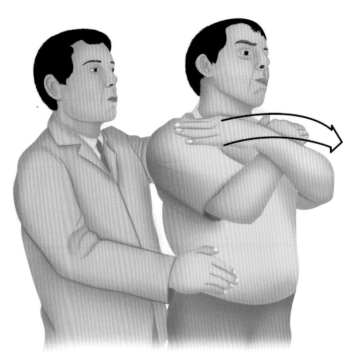

Fig. 4.9 Passive rotation.

Side Bending

To test resisted side bending, sit next to the seated patient. Wrap one arm around the patient's back and place your other hand on the patient's shoulder (**Fig. 4.12**). Sit close to the patient, and place the lateral side of your pelvis against the patient's pelvis to lock it into place. Instruct the patient to side bend away from you, and resist the motion. Note any weakness or pain.

■ Tests

Straight Leg Raise

To perform the straight leg raise, instruct the patient to lie supine on the exam table. With one hand, take hold of the patient's leg just above the malleoli; place the other hand on the thigh just above the knee. Raise the leg with the knee extended (**Fig. 4.13**). Stop flexing the hip when pain is felt in the back and leg. Be sure to differentiate radicular (pain in the distribution of a dermatome) leg pain from tight hamstrings. A true-positive straight leg-raising test is one that re-creates the patient's radicular pain and not just back pain.

Bragard's Test

Begin the Bragard's test by performing the straight leg raise. When the leg reaches the painful level of hip flexion, stop and slightly lower the leg until the pain has resolved. Hold the leg in this position, then remove the hand on the thigh and grasp the foot. Bring the foot into dorsiflexion (**Fig. 4.14**). If the symptom is reproduced, dural irritation is indicated.

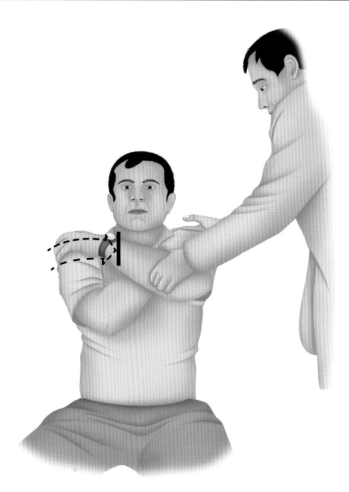

Fig. 4.10 Resisted rotation.

Neri's Test

To perform the Neri's test, begin by performing the straight leg raise. When the leg reaches the painful level of hip flexion, stop and slightly lower the leg until the pain has resolved (**Fig. 4.14**). Ask the patient to flex the neck and bring the chin to the chest. If pain is again provoked, dural irritation is indicated.

Combination Bragard's and Neri's Test

The Bragard's and Neri's tests can be used in combination with the straight leg raise to further stretch the dura mater. Raise the patient's extended leg. Instruct the patient to flex the neck as you bring the foot into dorsiflexion (**Fig. 4.14**). The dura is then maximally stretched; pain indicates dural irritation.

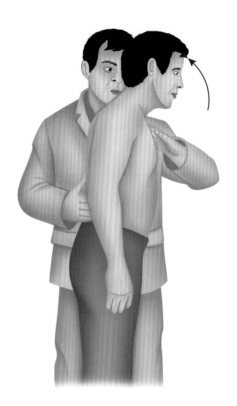

Fig. 4.11 Resisted flexion.

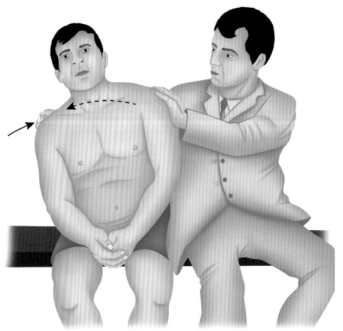

Fig. 4.12 Resisted side bending.

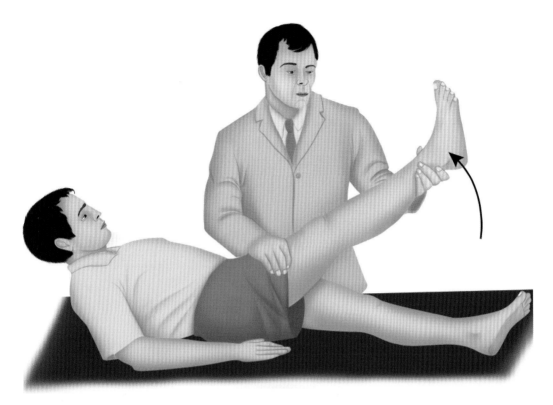

Fig. 4.13 Straight leg raising is performed with the patient lying supine on the table. The test is stopped when pain is felt. A true-positive straight leg-raising test re-creates the patient's radicular pain.

■ Neurologic Evaluation of the Lumbar Spine: L1–L3

Muscle Testing

L1, L2, and L3 are tested in combination due to a lack of specific muscle testing. The muscles commonly tested are the iliopsoas, the quadriceps, and the hip adductors (**Fig. 4.15**).

Hip Flexion

To test hip flexion, instruct the patient to sit on the edge of the examination table. Stand next to the patient, and place one hand on the patient's thigh just above the knee (**Fig. 4.16**).

Place your other hand on the patient's shoulder. Ask the patient to raise the knee against the resistance. This test should be repeated on the other side. A difference in strength between the two sides or other abnormalities should be noted.

- Muscle
  - Iliopsoas

- Innervation
  - Nerve roots (T12, L1, L2, L3)

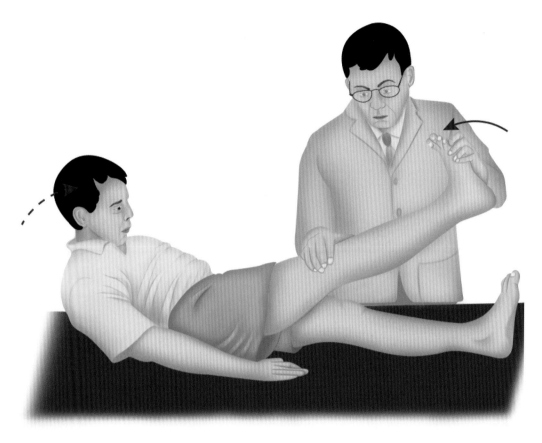

Fig. 4.14 The Bragard's test. Slightly lower the patient's leg after pain is produced, and dorsiflex the foot. The Neri's test is performed similarly, lowering the patient's leg after pain is produced and having the patient flex their neck, bringing the chin to the chest. If pain is provoked, dural irritation is indicated.

Knee Extension

To test knee extension, instruct the patient to sit on the examination table with the knees bent at 90 degrees and feet hanging toward the floor. Place one hand on the patient's thigh and the other on the distal leg. Ask the patient to fully extend the leg. When the leg is fully extended, try to forcefully flex the leg. Compare the legs (**Fig. 4.17**).

- Muscle
  - Quadriceps

- Innervation
  - Femoral nerve (L2, L3, L4)

Hip Adduction

To test hip adduction, instruct the patient to lie supine on the examination table and abduct the legs. Place your hands on the medial aspects of the knees, and ask the patient to bring the legs together in adduction (**Fig. 4.18**).

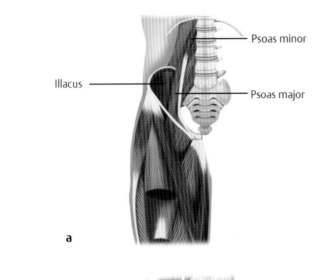

Illacus

Psoas minor

Psoas major

a

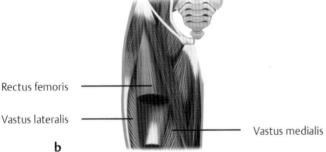

Rectus femoris

Vastus lateralis

Vastus medialis

b

Fig. 4.15 (**a**) Iliopsoas musculature innervated by T12, L1, L2, and L3. (**b**) Quadriceps musculature innervated by the femoral nerve (L2, L3, and L4).

- Muscles
  - Adductor brevis, adductor longus, adductor magnus

- Innervation
  - Obturator nerve (L2, L3, L4)

Reflex

Cremaster Reflex (T12, L1)

The cremaster reflex is an upper motor neuron reflex of males controlled by the cerebral cortex. A bilateral loss of the reflex indicates an upper motor neuron lesion above T12. A unilateral loss of the cremaster reflex may indicate a lower motor neuron lesion, most commonly between L1 and L2. To test the cremaster reflex, instruct the patient to undress below the waist. Gently stroke the medial aspect of the upper thigh with a fairly sharp object like the handle of the reflex hammer (**Fig. 4.19**). The scrotal sac on that side should elevate with contraction of the cremaster muscle.

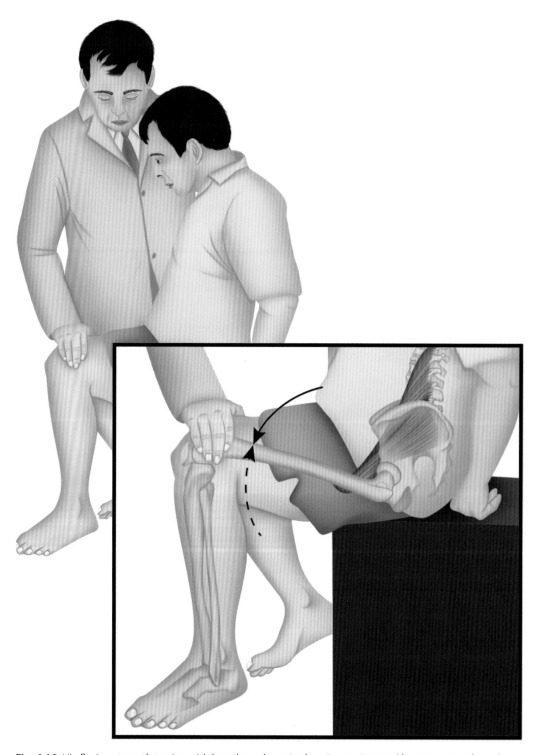

Fig. 4.16 Hip flexion strength testing with knee bent, leg raised against resistance (iliopsoas musculature).

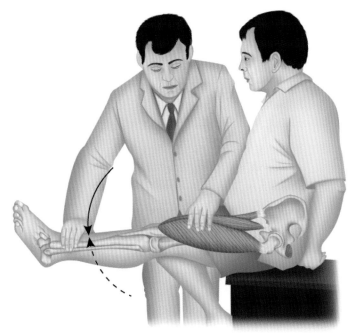

Fig. 4.17 Testing knee extension strength to evaluate quadriceps function.

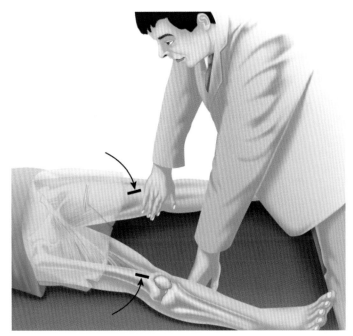

Fig. 4.18 Testing hip adduction (L2, L3, and 4).

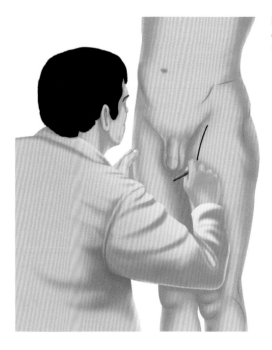

Fig. 4.19 Cremasteric reflex at T12, L1. Unilateral loss of the cremaster reflex may indicate a lower motor neuron lesion, commonly between L1 and L2.

Sensory

Sensory L1

Groin (**Fig. 4.20**).

Sensory L2

Lateral groin and anterior aspect of the thigh.

Sensory L3

Anteromedial aspect of the thigh to the malleoli.

■ Neurologic Evaluation of the Lumbar Spine: L4

Motor

Knee Extension

See LI–L3, above.

Dorsiflexion

To test dorsiflexion of the foot, instruct the patient to sit on the edge of the examination table. Take hold of the patient's distal leg superior to the malleoli. Ask the patient to dorsiflex and invert the foot. With your other hand, try to force the foot into plantar flexion and eversion (**Fig. 4.21**). Compare the tibialis anterior muscles. Asking the patient to walk on the heels is also a useful test of L4 motor function.

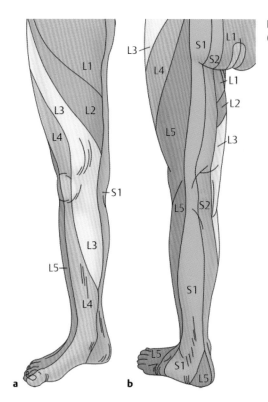

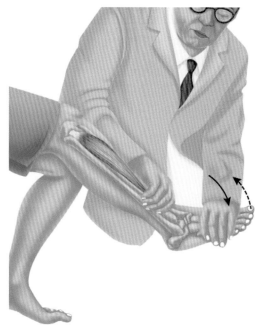

Fig. 4.20 (a) Dermatomes between L1 and S1. **(b)** Dermatomes between L1 and S2.

Fig. 4.21 Motor testing of the tibialis anterior (L4, L5).

- Muscle
  - Tibialis anterior

- Innervation
  - L4, L5

Reflex

Patellar Tendon Reflex (L4)

To test the patellar tendon reflex, instruct the patient to sit on the examination table with the quadriceps completely relaxed and legs dangling. With the reflex hammer, gently strike the patellar tendon just below the patella (**Fig. 4.22**). This should cause the quadriceps to contract and the knee to jerk. Compare the reflexes of the two legs.

Sensory

Sensory L4

Anterolateral aspect of the thigh and leg to the medial aspect of the great toe (**Fig. 4.23**).

■ Neurologic Evaluation of the Lumbar Spine: L5

Motor

Great Toe Extension

To test great toe extension, instruct the patient to sit on the examination table and extend the leg. With one hand, take hold of the leg just proximal to the malleoli. Place the index finger or

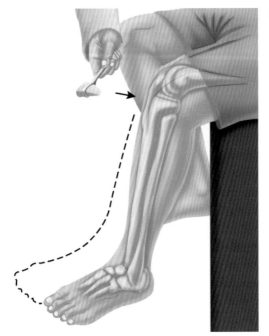

Fig. 4.22 Patellar tendon reflex (L4).

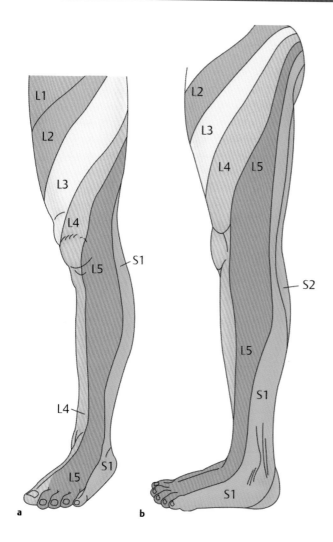

Fig. 4.23 (**a**) Dermatomal distribution in the lower extremity, L1 through S1. (**b**) Dermatomal distribution in the lower extremity, L1 through S2

thumb of your other hand on the interphalangeal joint of the big toe. Ask the patient to extend the toe while resistance is applied (**Fig. 4.24**).

- Muscle
  - Extensor hallucis longus

- Innervation
  - Deep peroneal nerve (L4, L5)

Hip Abduction

To test hip abduction, instruct the patient to lie on their side. Stabilize the hip with one hand, and place the other on the patient's knee. Ask the patient to raise the leg into abduction while resistance is applied (**Fig. 4.25**).

- Muscle
  - Gluteus medius

- Innervation
  - Superior gluteal nerve (L5)

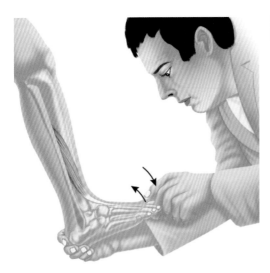

Fig. 4.24 Motor testing of the extensor hallucis longus (L5).

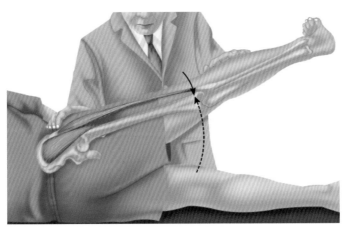

Fig. 4.25 Hip abduction strength tested with patient on side, raising the extended leg against resistance. This tests the gluteus medius muscle, innervated by L5 (superior gluteal nerve).

Reflex

Posterior Tibial Jerk

To elicit the posterior tibial jerk reflex, grasp the patient's foot and hold it in slight eversion and dorsiflexion. With the reflex hammer, strike the tendon of the tibialis posterior muscle just proximal to its insertion on the navicular tuberosity (**Fig. 4.26**). Stimulation of the reflex should result in a plantar inversion of the foot.

Sensory

Sensory L5

Posterior aspect of the thigh and lower leg, lateral aspect of the great toe, second toe, third toe, and the medial aspect of the fourth toe (**Fig. 4.23**).

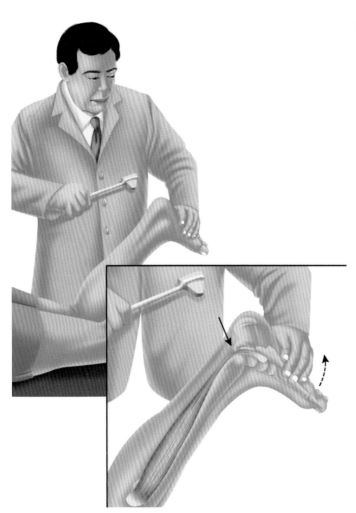

Fig. 4.26 Posterior tibial jerk (L5).

■ Neurologic Evaluation of the Sacral Spine: S1

Motor

Plantar Flexion

With the patient seated, grasp and secure the medial side of the patient's foot by fixing the calcaneus. Ask the patient to evert and plantar flex the foot. Resist the motion by using the fifth metatarsal (**Fig. 4.27**). Asking the patient to walk on tiptoes is also effective at testing S1 motor function.

- Muscles
    - Peroneus longus and peroneus brevis, gastrocnemius–soleus complex

- Innervation
    - Superficial peroneal nerve (S1)

Hip Extension

To test hip extension, instruct the patient to lie prone on the examination table and flex the knee of the side being tested. Place one hand on the iliac crest for stabilization and the other hand on the posterior aspect of the thigh. Ask the patient to raise the thigh off the table as you oppose the motion (**Fig. 4.28**). Compare the two sides.

- Muscle
  - Gluteus maximus

- Innervation
  - Inferior gluteal nerve (S1)

Reflex

Calcaneal Tendon Reflex

To elicit the calcaneal tendon reflex, instruct the patient to sit on the edge of the examination table with legs bent, dangling, and relaxed. Place the foot into slight dorsiflexion. Find the calcaneal tendon, and gently strike it with the reflex hammer (**Fig. 4.29**). This should elicit a plantar-directed jerk.

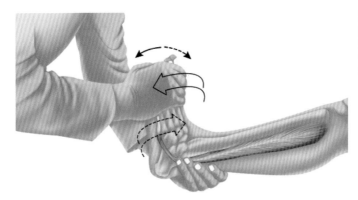

Fig. 4.27 Testing plantar flexion strength (S1). Having the patient walk on tiptoes is also a useful motor test for the gastrocnemius–soleus complex.

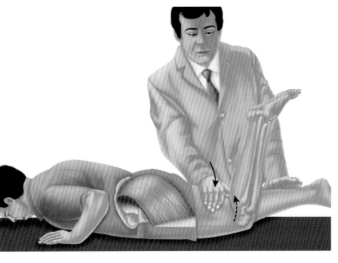

Fig. 4.28 Hip extension testing the gluteus maximus (S1).

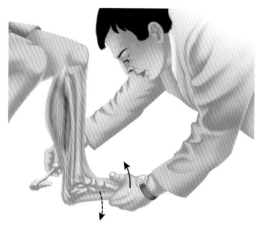

Fig. 4.29 Calcaneal tendon reflex (S1).

Sensory

Posterior aspect of the thigh and lower leg, lateral aspect of the foot, lateral-most aspect of the fourth toe, and the fifth toe (**Fig. 4.23**).

■ Neurologic Levels S2, S3, and S4

Motor

S2, S3, and S4 innervate the intrinsic muscles of the feet and the anal sphincter. Inspect each foot, and look for deformities of the toes. The bladder is also innervated by these nerve roots, so questions about bladder function should be included when taking the patient's history.

External Anal Sphincter (S4, S5)

To test the external anal sphincter, instruct the patient to undress below the waist. The patient lies on their side and brings the hips and knees into flexion. Instruct the patient to relax, and insert a gloved and lubricated finger into the rectum. Ask the patient to contract the anal sphincter, and feel for a change in sphincter tone (**Fig. 4.30**).

Reflex

Babinski's Sign (S2, S3)

To perform the Babinski's test, take the patient's foot with one hand. Using the handle of the reflex hammer or a sharp object, stroke the bottom of the foot. Starting at the heel, pull the handle of the reflex hammer along the lateral plantar surface of the foot.

   When the tuberosity of the fifth metatarsal is reached, turn and stroke in a medial direction toward the tuberosity of the big toe (**Fig. 4.31**). Proper initiation of the reflex may require a strong and forceful stroke. The test is positive if the big toe extends. A positive Babinski's sign indicates an upper motor neuron lesion. It should be included as a test to rule out cervical and/or thoracic myelopathy in all spinal examinations.

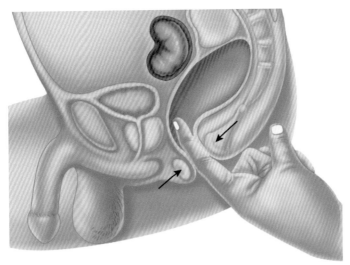

Fig. 4.30 Checking the external anal sphincter (S4, S5) for sphincter tone. Ask the patient to contract the sphincter.

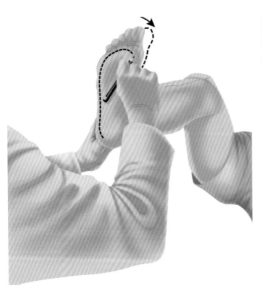

Fig. 4.31 Babinski's sign (S2, S3). The test is positive if the big toe extends, indicating an upper motor neuron lesion. Normally the toes curl downward with this maneuver.

Oppenheim's Test

To perform the Oppenheim's test, run a sharp object, or your index finger and thumb, downward while squeezing along the crest of the tibia (**Fig. 4.32**). If the big toe extends, the test is positive and indicates an upper motor neuron lesion.

Bulbocavernosus Reflex (S2, S3, S4)

To elicit the bulbocavernosus reflex, instruct the patient to undress below the waist. The patient lies on their side and brings the hips and knees into flexion. Instruct the patient to relax, and insert a gloved and lubricated finger into the rectum. With the other hand, squeeze the penis or clitoris (**Fig. 4.33**). The gloved finger in the rectum should feel the contraction of the anal sphincter.

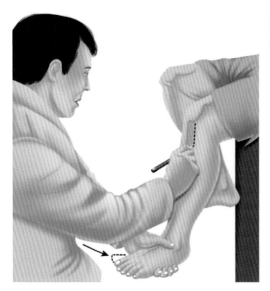

Fig. 4.32 Oppenheim's test, similar to Babinski's test, but elicited by running a sharp object down the pretibial area along the crest of the tibia.

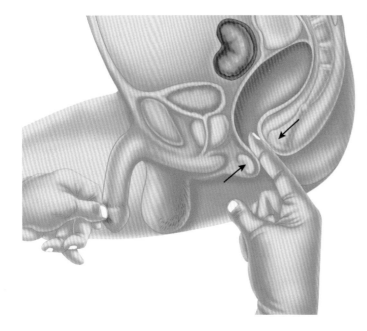

Fig. 4.33 Testing the bulbocavernosus reflex (S2, S3, S4) with the finger in the rectum. When the penis or clitoris is squeezed, there should be a contraction of the anal sphincter, indicating an intact reflex. Absence of the reflex can indicate spinal shock after a traumatic episode.

Anocutaneous Reflex (S3, S4, S5)

To elicit the anocutaneous reflex, instruct the patient to lie supine on the examination table and flex both hips so that the thighs and legs form an angle of 90 degrees with the trunk. With a pin, stimulate the sensory dermatomes of S3, S4, and S5, and watch for contraction of the anal sphincter (**Fig. 4.34**).

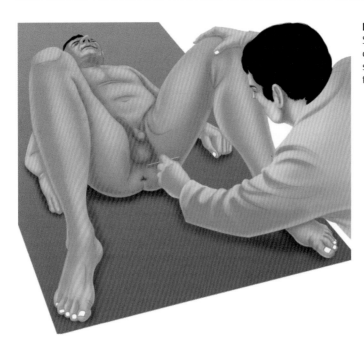

Fig. 4.34 Anocutaneous reflex (S3, S4, S5). Stimulating the sensory dermatomes of S3, S4, and S5 should produce a contraction of the anal sphincter (anal wink).

Sensory

Sensory S2

Posterior aspect of the thigh and lower leg, including the plantar aspect of the heel.

Sensory S3

Medial aspect of the thigh.

Sensory S4

Perineum.

Sensory S5

Perianal region.

Index